Sheldon Mii
Anxiety and I

Dr Cheryl Rezek is a consultant clinical psychologist and mindfulness teacher who brings a fresh and dynamic approach to how mindfulness and psychological concepts can be integrated into everyone's life as a way of managing it in the most helpful way. Her work is engaging, accessible and, most importantly, realistic, and her writing easy to read and follow, giving it a broad appeal to all audiences. Her model (affectionately known as Life Happens) is based on academic knowledge and her extensive clinical experience, and it is regarded as an emerging mindfulness-based approach. It encourages awareness of oneself within a context, the development of resilience and skills, and the use of mindfulness. She has a long-standing clinical and academic career; she's lectured, supervised, developed programmes, appeared on radio and TV shows, as well as run workshops nationally and internationally. She is the author of a number of books, including *Life Happens: Waking up to yourself and your life in a mindful way* (Leachcroft); *Mindfulness: How the mindful approach can help you towards a better life* (Pearson); *Mindfulness for Carers: How to manage the demands of caregiving while finding a place for yourself* (Jessica Kingsley); *Monkey Mind and the Mountain: Mindfulness for 8–12-year-olds (and older)* (Leachcroft); and *Sheldon Mindfulness: Quit Smoking* (Sheldon Press). Dr Rezek also has a highly rated app entitled *iMindfulness on the Go* (Android and iOS).

Visit her website at <www.lifehappens-mindfulness.com>.

4 1 0256746 0

Sheldon Mindfulness

Selected titles

A full list of titles is available from Sheldon Press,
36 Causton Street, London SW1P 4ST and on our website at
www.sheldonpress.co.uk

Sheldon Mindfulness

Anxiety and Depression

DR CHERYL REZEK

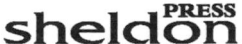

First published in Great Britain in 2016

Sheldon Press
36 Causton Street
London SW1P 4ST
www.sheldonpress.co.uk

The author and publisher have made every effort to ensure that the
external website and email addresses included in this book are correct
and up to date at the time of going to press. The author and publisher
are not responsible for the content, quality or continuing accessibility of
the sites.

British Library Cataloguing-in-Publication Data
A catalogue record for this book is available from the British Library

ISBN 978–1–84709–417–9
eBook ISBN 978–1–84709–418–6

Typeset by Fakenham Prepress Solutions, Fakenham, Norfolk NR21 8NN
First printed in Great Britain by Ashford Colour Press
Subsequently digitally reprinted in Great Britain

eBook by Fakenham Prepress Solutions, Fakenham, Norfolk NR21 8NN

Produced on paper from sustainable forests

Many thanks to Emmy Fisher for her assistance with this project.

Contents

An important note about the text

To access the audio downloads that accompany this book, go to: <www.lifehappens-mindfulness.com/book-audio>.

Do not listen to the audio download material while driving or operating any machinery or item.

Disclaimer: This book makes no claim to act as a cure or treatment for any conditions, nor does it advocate discontinuation of any intervention or treatment.

Introduction

Life happens

Life happens for better and for worse. It gives us both our most cherished moments and experiences that throw us into turmoil and chaos. At times when we feel anxious or depressed, it can be very difficult to see how life could be different. If you have ever felt that life is just one struggle after the next, felt a sense of panic about where your life is heading, or just tried to block out the present in order to suppress your anxiety and distress, then a mindful approach can help you build resilience and cultivate an inner calmness and stability.

Mindfulness is an approach that can help reconcile all the joys and challenges of your life, enabling you to choose how you want to be within each moment, to live out your life in a balanced and considered way.

How to use this book

This book provides an introduction to mindfulness, the concepts and theory behind it and the way it has been adapted into an approach that has been used to manage not only anxiety but a number of physical and emotional issues. Importantly, by combining it with key psychological concepts and skills, it provides you with an integrated, useful casket of treasure. Step-by-step it leads you through how this approach can be used to manage your anxiety and depression and be implemented into your life by developing an understanding of yourself, your situation and a mindful approach to life. Engaging with the ideas and practices that are included, both in written form and in an audio download of guided meditations, will help you reap the rewards.

> To download the guided meditations, go to <www.lifehappens-mind fulness/book-audio>. Whenever you see this symbol ◀)) it indicates that there is a guided meditation in the form of an audio download that you can listen to.

Mindfulness is an approach to life, so it can be used without the practices spread throughout this book. However, the practices are the cornerstone to mindfulness work and are an invaluable tool for managing anxiety or depression. At times you may be reluctant to listen to the audio download material as you won't know what to expect, so short transcripts of parts of them have been made available in this book. Making time to do the practices will transfer the theories and ideas into a practical and helpful tool that you can use throughout your life.

Each part is important in its own right, so try to find one aspect of each that interests or engages you the most. This will motivate you to continue with the suggestions and practices, which will have a positive impact on your sense of balance and well-being and help to transform your life. If you want the benefits you do need to do the work. Nothing can happen if you don't.

At the end of each chapter there is a blank page entitled 'Notes to myself'. Use these pages as a way of keeping a running commentary or journal to yourself on anything that comes to mind as you move through the book. You can also use them as a mindfulness journal, to recognize how mindfulness is impacting on you as you work through the chapters.

Part 1

Understanding anxiety, depression and mindfulness

1

Connecting the dots

Making sense of your life

This book combines the age-old philosophies of mindfulness with the research and clinical meaning of psychology in everyday life, to help you examine your life and your anxieties in a thoughtful way. It makes no claim to change your life, but it is a resource that can be developed to provide you with a sense of balance and calm on which to draw when life is at its most chaotic and destructive. It can also enable you to be fully present in moments of happiness and peace, promoting your emotional, mental and physical health and well-being. By taking the time to do the practices and paying attention to your life, you will find that you are more able to make sense of your life and recognize positive choices, which will bring a feeling of being grounded and stable.

When we feel depressed or our levels of anxiety and stress are high, it is difficult to see how life can be any different or anticipate a time when we will feel more in control and happy. Feelings of emotional distress often develop over a long period and for a number of different reasons. Giving yourself the time to think about how you are feeling can help you understand your past experiences and make the links to your emotions and reactions in the present.

Once you begin to connect the dots, it becomes much easier to see the bigger picture and make thoughtful, mindful decisions about how to live your life.

Understanding anxiety and depression

One in four people will meet the criteria for an anxiety disorder, mood disorder or alcohol dependence at some time in their life, and mixed anxiety and depression is the most common mental health issue in the UK, where approximately 9 per cent of adults would meet the criteria for diagnosis at any time.[1] Although this figure is high, it is unsurprising given the constant demands and pressures of modern life. You don't need to be diagnosed with an anxiety disorder or depression to know that you are experiencing symptoms of them, and there is no shame in admitting to yourself that you are unhappy with your life or would like to engage with it in a more open way.

Everyone experiences times when life seems difficult or overwhelming.

This part of the book explores what anxiety and depression are in more detail; if you are experiencing any of these symptoms, then mindfulness practice may be very beneficial for you. Although anxiety and depression are often considered separately, many people have symptoms of both. During times of stress or when feeling overwhelmed, it isn't uncommon to experience low mood or lose confidence in yourself. Likewise, when you feel depressed and your self-esteem is low, you can feel uneasy about social situations or start to panic when emotions build up.

Notes to myself

2

Anxiety, depression and mindfulness

What is anxiety?

Anxiety can take many forms – it may be a specific phobia, such as of heights or small spaces, a fear of social embarrassment or humiliation, a general feeling of unease or nervousness, or a feeling of panic and being overwhelmed. Perhaps some of the following physical, psychological or emotional symptoms will seem familiar:

- nausea or stomach pain
- sweating
- headache or migraine
- breathlessness and chest pain
- palpitations
- fast heart rate
- muscle tension
- shaking
- dry mouth
- low mood
- irritability
- restlessness
- disturbed sleep or insomnia
- poor concentration
- recurring thoughts

- feelings of apprehension or dread
- nervousness and feeling jittery
- increased use of alcohol or drugs
- phobias
- panic attacks.

Whatever its form, anxiety can affect your mood, your relationships and your well-being, and it is a sign that you need to intervene in your life.

Fear is an emotional and physical response to things that you perceive to have the potential to harm you. At a basic level it triggers the 'fight or flight' response, which is a primitive, automatic, reaction at an evolutionary level, allowing you to react quickly to protect you from whatever is threatening you.[1] However, when fear occurs in anticipation of something that you think is a threat but isn't (a perceived threat, such as from being stuck in traffic), or when no threat is present, then it can become problematic. This is the essence of anxiety – a feeling of apprehension or nervousness that occurs when there is no immediate threat present to cause or justify it.

Most people have experienced anxiety at some time in their life – feelings of fear and apprehension are normal responses. However, when these feelings begin to interfere with your life on a frequent basis and restrict the things you feel you are able to do, then they ought to be addressed.

What is depression?

Depression affects your thoughts, feelings and involvement in your life. It may cause you to be low in mood, tearful, despairing, restless or agitated. Alternatively, people with depression may feel numb or empty inside. Depression can affect how you relate to other people, and you may find yourself cutting yourself off from others or being unable to ask for help. People who have depression generally have low self-confidence and may think they are not good enough or feel guilty a lot of the time. During times of depression, people tend to feel that their future is bleak and find it difficult to imagine a time when life will feel happier and easier. It may cause the following symptoms, among others:

- persistent low mood
- feelings of despair or hopelessness
- helplessness
- difficulty making decisions
- speaking or moving more slowly
- irritability
- tearfulness
- lack of energy
- decreased interest in sex
- emotional numbness
- low self-esteem
- increased use of painkillers
- disturbed sleep
- changes in weight and appetite
- aches and pains
- increased alcohol and drug use
- thoughts of harming yourself
- loss of interest in activities you enjoy.

Everyone experiences fluctuations in mood, and it is unrealistic to think that you can feel fantastic every moment of every day. When low moods become persistent, however, and they are accompanied by other symptoms of depression, these feelings need to be dealt with to reduce the negative effects they may have on your life, and contain any urges to harm yourself or others as well as increase your happiness and well-being.

Mindfulness practice: A Moment of Stillness

This exercise is a simple but effective way to begin to understand what mindfulness is about. It can be used as a starting point or as a marker of your progress as you become more involved in the process of mindfulness.

- Sit in stillness for two minutes.
- Pay attention to what thoughts and sensations are going through your mind. Is there an itch in your leg? Have you just remembered that you need to pay the phone bill? Do your shoulders feel tense? Is your heart pounding? Are you thinking about all the things on your to-do list?

What was it like sitting in stillness – did you feel comfortable or were you in any physical or emotional discomfort? Did you start to feel calmer or did your anxiety start to increase? Did the time go quickly or slowly? Why do you think that was?

When you take the time to sit in stillness, often your mind can be overrun by all the things queuing for your attention. This is especially true for people who have high levels of anxiety – the prospect of stopping for one moment and letting these thoughts come and go can be daunting. The mindfulness practices in this book can help you develop your focus, allowing you to take a step back from these thoughts and feelings and gently quieten your anxieties and distress.

A mindful approach

Mindfulness is about paying attention to, and accepting, your thoughts, feelings and responses to cultivate an alert and balanced state of mind.

- It is an approach to life that involves both practices and the development of a way of being, a mindset.
- It can be developed and used by anyone and everyone.
- It is about relearning the ability that you had as a child to accept the present moment and to only be in this moment.

- It is not relaxation or an altered state of mind.
- It is a resource you can draw on in difficult times and a way to fully enjoy the good times.

When we are anxious or depressed it is often easiest to bury our heads in the sand, hide away or else distract ourselves from our fears with alcohol, drugs and other negative behaviours. A mindful approach to life is one that encourages kindness and understanding towards yourself, providing a safe and stable anchor to each and every moment. It is not a cure or treatment but a way of life that promotes resilience, no matter what life may throw at us.

A brief history of mindfulness

Mindfulness is a key component of Buddhist and other philosophies, which stretch back over two and a half thousand years.[2] Meditations focusing on breathing and being present in the moment are an important part of Buddhist practices, and their effectiveness and usefulness have filtered through to the Western world over the centuries. In 1979, colleagues at the University of Massachusetts developed a programme that integrated these mindfulness practices into a structured format to provide interventions for people suffering from physical and emotional distress in a hospital setting. This programme became known as Mindfulness-Based Stress Reduction (MBSR), which is now an internationally recognized programme that has been used worldwide for a variety of physical and emotional conditions.

Focused attention

Meditation is a term that often invokes the idea of a trance-like state, of zoning out of your surroundings and retreating into your mind or of seeking some elevated state of enlightenment. However, within the context of mindfulness it refers to paying attention to the present moment, for whatever it brings. By focusing on your breathing, the most automatic of functions, in this moment without evaluating or judging it, you are able to appreciate and absorb the moment for what it is – the sensations in your body, the sights, sounds and smells around you, the emotions you are experiencing – in a stable, balanced and non-reactive way. Instead of zoning out, mindfulness meditation brings your awareness to your life right now, grounding you and allowing you to be alive to this moment of your life.

Mindfulness is about switching on, not switching off.

Mindfulness practice: Mindful Eating

- Take a piece of fruit, chocolate or any other food that is not too difficult to chew.
- Eat one piece as normal.
- Now take another piece, place it on your tongue and let it sit there for a few moments.
- Bring all your attention to the sensation in your mouth as you let the food remain there without chewing or swallowing it. What does it feel like in your mouth – rough or smooth? What does it taste like, and can you identify any elements to the taste you hadn't noticed with the previous piece?
- Chew the food slowly. What other sensations do you feel? Is it difficult to resist the urge to swallow?
- Now swallow and notice the movements that come with this action.

Notes to myself

3

Facts, figures and you

The World Health Organization (WHO) reports that globally 350 million people of all ages suffer from depression and about 450 million from a mental health disorder.[1]

- Depression is the leading cause of disability worldwide, across high-, middle- and low-income countries.
- It is a major contributor to the global burden of disease.
- More women than men suffer from depression (1:4 versus 1:10 in the population).
- Depression leads to one million deaths per year from suicide.
- Suicide is the second leading cause of death among 15–29-year-olds worldwide but is the *main* cause of death in this age group in many European countries.
- There is a higher rate of suicide among men than women as more women attempt suicide than men but more men succeed (except in rural China, where more women commit suicide than men).
- Suicide attempts are 20–25 times higher than suicide rates.
- Some 75 per cent of suicides globally occur in low- and middle-income countries.
- The UK has one of the highest rates of self-harm in Europe.[2]

It is estimated around 17 per cent of the US population will suffer from a major depressive episode at least once in their lifetime; 27 per cent of adults in the USA will experience mental health problems in any 12-month period.[3] In the UK, 8–12 per cent of the population will experience depression in any 12-month period and around 1 in 4 UK adults will have at least one diagnosable mental health problem in the same period.[4]

According to the Mental Health Foundation, in the UK:

- women are twice as likely as men to experience anxiety;
- women make up around 60 per cent of those with a phobia or obsessive compulsive disorder (OCD);
- Generalized Anxiety Disorder (GAD) affects around 2–5 per cent of the population but up to 30 per cent of GP visits in the UK are due to this condition;
- while 2.6 per cent of the population experience depression and 4.7 per cent anxiety, as many as 9.7 per cent suffer from mixed depression and anxiety, which makes it the most prevalent mental health problem in the population as a whole;
- in the UK, 1 in 5 people report feeling anxious all the time;
- one-fifth of people who experience anxiety never seek help or attempt to do anything about it;
- a little under half of those who get anxious report that they are more anxious now than in previous times and that anxiety has stopped them from doing things.[5]

In the USA:

- anxiety is the most common mental illness, affecting 40 million from the age of 18, which is approximately 18 per cent of the population;
- it costs the USA more than $42 billion a year, which is approximately a third of the country's mental health bill of $148 billion;
- more than $22 billion of the cost is due to people with anxiety disorders seeking help for symptoms that mimic physical illnesses, such as shortness of breath;
- people with anxiety disorders are 3–5 times more likely to go to the doctor and 6 times more likely to be admitted to hospital for psychiatric disorders than those without an anxiety disorder.[6]

Anxiety and depression in older adults (aged 60 and above)

This population group is estimated to double from 11 per cent to 22 per cent worldwide between the years 2000 and 2050, and treble by 2100. It is thought that 15 per cent of people 60 or above suffer from a mental disorder, 20 per cent from a mental or neurological disorder and 6.6 per cent from a mental health and neurological disorder.[7]

- Anxiety disorders affect 3.8 per cent.
- Substance misuse almost 1 per cent.
- A quarter of deaths from self-harm are people from this age group.
- Depression affects 1 in 5 older adults living in the community and 2 in 5 living in care homes.
- In the USA there is 1 suicide for every estimated 4 suicide attempts in the elderly.[8]
- Globally, women over 70 are twice as likely to die from suicide than women aged 15–29.
- Suicides among men are the highest in those over 75.[9]

This age group is frequently under-diagnosed and under-treated for mental health problems, partly due to care professionals not looking out for it, combined with their thinking that low mood or feelings of anxiety or fear come with getting older. Added to this is the fact that professionals are often embarrassed or reticent to put sensitive questions to older adults or don't think that issues of alcohol abuse or sexual abuse really figure among this age group. This is a serious concern as this age group are also more vulnerable to mental health difficulties due to factors such as loneliness, less independence, substance abuse and being sexually, physically or emotionally abused, including by family, neighbours or care staff.[10] In addition to this, it is known that mental health impacts on physical health and that people with physical conditions, especially if chronic (such as cardiovascular disease, diabetes, psoriasis, pain conditions and others), have a much higher risk of developing depression than those who are healthy.

Untreated depression impacts negatively on physical disease, and low mood influences levels of pain, motivation to attend treatments and even healing and recovery after surgery.[11]

Workplace

In 2013–14, work-related stress, depression or anxiety cases in the UK made up 39 per cent of all work-related illnesses.[12] The loss on average per case of stress, depression or anxiety was 23 days, which then resulted in these conditions accumulating to a total loss of a staggering 11.3 million days in 2013–14. A report in 2012 estimated that the direct costs of absence alone amounted to over £14 billion across the economy in the UK, non-work-related mental health issues being one of the three major contributors, the others back pain and musculoskeletal disorders. Non-work-related mental health issues are most commonly identified as causing long-term absence.[13]

Suicide

As previously noted, around one million people die from suicide each year. Of great concern is that suicide is the most common cause of death in men under the age of 35. It used to be men in the 18–24 age range who where most at risk but in recent years there has been a shift towards men in older age ranges.

In the USA:

- 38,000 people die from suicide every year;
- the highest number is from the 20–24 age range;[14]
- from 1999 to 2010, suicide rates for those aged 35–64 rose by almost 30 per cent;
- the most pronounced increase was seen in men in their fifties, where a 50 per cent increase was found;
- suicide rates are growing among both middle-aged men and middle-aged women.[15,16]

In the UK:

- 6,233 suicides of people aged 15 and over were registered in the UK in 2013, whereas only 5,981 were registered in 2012;
- this meant that 252 more people killed themselves than in 2012 (around a 4 per cent increase);
- the male suicide rate in 2013 was the highest since 2001;
- the age range with the highest UK suicide rate in 2012 was men aged 40–45 but in 2013 it was men aged 45–59 (which fits with people aged 50–54 having showed the highest rates of depression in 2013);
- men are almost 4 times more likely to commit suicide than women;
- the suicide rate in prisons is around 15 times higher than in the general population, and men in prison are 14 times more likely to have a mental disorder than men in general and women 35 times more so than women in general.[17,18]

People get anxious and depressed for different reasons, which fall within general categories of biological, psychological and social, so there is seldom only a single cause. Not all people who are depressed commit suicide, which tends to happen in moments of crisis, under life stressors such as financial problems, relationship breakdowns, isolation, when using substances, having an illness or being in chronic pain.[19] The World Health Organization also reports that experiencing conflict, disaster, violence, abuse or loss, and a sense of isolation, are strongly associated with suicidal behaviour.

What should also be kept in mind is that suicide rates are high among vulnerable groups, such as those who experience discrimination. For example:

- minority ethnic groups
- lesbian, gay, bisexual, transgender and intersex persons
- prisoners
- refugees and migrants.[20]

Stigma

The stigma of having depressed, anxious or difficult feelings is one of the primary reasons people hold back from speaking about their problems and from seeking help. This can be in a work setting but extends far beyond that to families, and can be affected by cultural taboos and religious beliefs. Many cases of suicide, for example, go unreported or the cause of death is put under a different category due to shame, fear of being ostracized or rejected by communities or religious organizations.[21]

People throughout the world fear ridicule, rejection or dismissal if they reveal their feelings, especially of distress. Sometimes they even run the risk of being imprisoned or persecuted if it's discovered that their distress is over, for example, being homosexual or revealing abuse. Persecution and dismissal can take subversive as well as more obvious forms.

The stigma of having a diagnosed condition is there too as it can frequently make people even more concerned as there is now a labelled mental health disorder rather than a set of symptoms.

Feelings and symptoms versus disorder

There are both advantages and disadvantages to labelling a set of symptoms as a disorder. The advantage is that people can feel a sense of relief knowing why they feel as they do. The term 'disorder' is a very unfortunate one, extensively used in the field of mental health and rooted in the medical model. It assists people to understand the range of symptoms that may come with their disorder and for professionals to know immediately what might be a reason for certain behaviours and symptoms, and it provides a sense of clarity and structure that can assist the individual, research teams and interventions so it does have a value. However, it can also be rigid and dehumanizing.

One of the biggest disadvantages of having a formal diagnosis of a disorder – and the emphasis is on the word 'disorder', such as major depressive *disorder* or generalized anxiety *disorder*, not the fact of having a condition – is that once a label has been placed on someone it is difficult to shift from it. It may create a sense of living within a box that then influences how you think about yourself. A further concern is that both the individual and the professionals around them tend to focus on the disorder label and its concurrent symptoms, rather than on the person, where these feelings and behaviours come from, how they developed and what the individual, you, can do for yourself to start addressing them. Labels run the risk of shifting some of the responsibility from you and what you need to be doing, to something that can become an external box.

In the light of stigma, the fear of being given a label of a disorder may discourage people from seeking help. 'I don't need to speak to anyone about my problems; I'm not mad' is commonly heard and is possibly a barrier that has been created by fear, different cultural attitudes and the media, who portray mental health concerns in such a distorted way.

What is being raised is not that there shouldn't be diagnoses, because that is essential and extremely important, but rather how such labels of disorders might affect people with them and those around them. If you are depressed and anxious, you are depressed and anxious, and those feelings are coming from within you, so you can begin to look at them. They don't belong to a pre-packaged disorder that is being placed upon you and therefore over which you have no control. By the same token, some people may want to hide behind the label and, consciously or unconsciously, have it there as a means of protecting themselves from addressing or facing what needs to be done.

This concept is particularly important, in fact fundamental, to any moving forward with your anxiety and depression, or any other condition. Mental health is more complicated than physical health because it can't be seen under a microscope or on an MRI scan. However, this doesn't mean that it can't be worked with. How you feel is a set of feelings, a range of emotions that influence your life.

You are not your depression or anxiety – it is part of you but not all of you, because you have many other facets to your personality and abilities.

It may profoundly influence what you think and do but depression, as such, doesn't make you feel bad about yourself or stop you from socializing, relating or working. It's to do with how you feel about yourself and the world, and that is a major factor in your becoming depressed. Not socializing because of your low mood or anxiety then adds to your feeling bad about yourself, which affects your sense of self-worth and esteem. The point being made is that depression is the result of how you view yourself and the world rather than of you having a disorder that then imposes this view upon you. You weren't born with depression or anxiety – it has developed for whatever reasons. You may have a predisposition to them, but – once more – that doesn't mean you would have automatically developed them. A predisposition implies only a greater possibility rather than a definite, and role modelling, family and social factors play a key part in pre-dispositions emerging into full-blown conditions.

Notes to myself

4

Men and depression

You may be wondering why there is a chapter on men and depression, and perhaps why there isn't therefore one on women too. The reason is because much of the research done on depression, anxiety and their symptoms is based on women. Women, on the whole, will far more readily identify what is happening to them by recognizing the symptoms, and will seek help or support either from friends and relatives or from professionals.

A serious concern is that men more often than not don't know the symptoms, and more importantly, even if they were to know them, men tend to show different symptoms from women. This poor recognition is pervasive among professionals too, so even if men did present to their doctors or other healthcare professionals with one set of symptoms, these wouldn't necessarily be identified as depression.

Men may display many of the traditionally recognized symptoms previously mentioned, but they may not. Some of the less obvious ones are:

- an increase in feelings of anger or aggression;
- being more aggressive either physically or verbally, even emotionally;
- being agitated;
- working excessive hours;
- an increase in the use of drugs or alcohol or any substance that alters mood;

- an increase in sexual activity or getting involved in reckless or unprotected sex, watching pornography or greater amounts of it;
- risk taking – this covers gambling, making financial deals you wouldn't normally make;
- being more impulsive and caring less about the consequences;
- an increase in exercise, beyond being on a specific training programme or for a particular purpose;
- feeling a need to protect yourself or close ranks around yourself; for example, reducing your social contacts to only one or two friends or spending increasing amounts of time on your own or in solitary pursuits;
- feeling heavy, trapped or restless.

In terms of anxiety, men and women tend to have the same symptoms, although these may vary depending on the individual.

Social training

Women are more exposed to feelings and trained from a very early age to recognize and put words to them. This emotional vocabulary is more readily available to them in times of need: in general they might have received a cuddle when feeling worried or low as a child, whereas a boy might have had his hair ruffled and been told to go out and play. Little girls will be engaged in conversations about their dolls and their doll's emotions – 'Have you fed her? She'll start crying if you don't; Is she crying? Why is she upset? Did somebody shout at her? Have you given her a hug?' These are not the lines of conversation you'll hear when a little boy has crashed his toy car into the furniture or is jumping off the edge of the sofa dressed as Spiderman. No one ventures to say 'Is Spiderman scared of heights? Do you think he's upset? Is he hungry? Did someone shout at him?'

For men, again in more general terms, the main acknowledgement of more difficult feelings is usually 'Boys don't cry. Don't be a baby. Toughen up. Are you a girl?' or something along those lines.

These attitudes are continually reinforced at many different levels, right from the start. The most obvious are parental attitudes and role modelling, which have a profound impact on children and their capacity to recognize and respond to their own feelings. They may become good at doing this for others and regard that as a positive quality, whereas doing it for themselves is something entirely different.

Culturally and socially there are few encouragements for men to learn that it is all right, first of all, to have feelings, and second, to express them. Even within a more liberal twenty-first-century Western culture, men either find the whole notion of emotional expression a bit at odds with their male image or dismiss it as something that is the domain of girls, not boys. Men will know what the words 'depression', 'anxiety', 'shame' and so forth mean, as words. The difficulty is being able to know what it is to be depressed; that is, what the symptoms are or what is associated with the word 'shame'. Women say the word and then add the explanations, and these are often added to by other women, so the dyad or group learn from each other and also familiarize themselves with the range and nuances of emotional states. This social or interactive learning is far less common among men. They often mock each other in a friendly way around those things called 'feelings'. The one emotion that seems to be excluded is anger. This is a more socially acceptable, and accepted, expression, which is perhaps why it is an important indicator of depression in men.

Some men do know what they are feeling but really struggle to seek help, believing it will make them appear weak or unable to cope. When a group of women are together they will talk, often either about emotions or their conversation will include something about how they feel, even if it's on a topic that isn't about feelings. Women attach feelings to conversations. Men, on the other hand, can stand next to each other or around a pub counter and converse in semi-silence. There will be no awkwardness. If there is a conversation, the tone is mostly different and attaching feelings to a topic wouldn't happen. It's about the quality or type of conversation that differs, rather than that words aren't being exchanged.

Language

Men are often put off by the type of language associated with emotions or personal issues. Phrases such as 'inner self', 'soul expression', 'emotional completeness' or 'getting in touch with feelings' do little to encourage men to look into what is happening. The language used in the areas or professions associated with therapeutic help is laden with vocabulary that is geared towards women or towards people who already know about emotional phraseology.

Fluffy language and little candles are not helpful.

Engaging men

Men are notoriously difficult to engage in discussions around health, whether physical or psychological. This is of enormous concern because men kill themselves, literally, or work hard at it through abusing substances, speeding, dangerous deals or activities, rather than speak to someone about what is happening. Speaking of difficult feelings is seen as an affront on masculinity, and asking for help a sure sign of weakness and of being unable to cope. It shakes their sense of status, of social competence and standing, and they fear those close to them, family, friends and colleagues, will think less of them, be embarrassed by their poor coping skills and lack of grit, and that they themselves will think the very same things.

Multiple angles

Perhaps there needs to be a multi-pronged approach to addressing these issues. On the one hand, the media can play an important role by running articles and programmes on men's psychological health, having interviews with high-profile men as well as with men from a variety of professions and walks of life – bankers, shopkeepers, coaches, waiters, retired men. Men need far greater exposure to hearing other men speak about their depression and anxiety and what helped them. These men and experts need to be on general talk shows, programmes and campaigns, not only specialist or dedicated ones, so that the whole notion of men struggling with life issues becomes familiar, open and accessible. If you can read, hear and see helpful, unsensationalized information on a poster, in an article, on the radio or in a TV talk show, you may pay attention to it because you don't then need to feel embarrassed or ashamed as it is being discussed openly. The other strand is for professionals to be more aware of the differences in how men show their depression and to be much more upfront by asking men how they feel. If a man does happen to go to the doctor for a physical complaint, a few well-chosen questions could make a big difference. It's essential that men are exposed to enough role modelling and information that tells them that it's all right to have feelings, to talk about them and to do something about them. The more exposure, the less stigmatizing and unfamiliar it can become.

The third prong to this is for you, men, to be willing to do something different. Working through this book will give a much better sense of what has and is happening in your life, and the mindfulness practices are a sound way of making time to stand still and think about it in a different way. If you are going to run, put your trainers on and mark out a route. If you're planning on using drugs, alcohol, sex, gambling, porn, aggressive video games or anything else to distract you from yourself, then know that some of them can become problems in themselves over time – and then you'll have two problems and not one.

Notes to myself

5

Your life

This is about your life

Society provides few resources for people who are struggling with life, and those that are available involve going from one assessment to another, with long waiting times and short interventions. There are alternatives that can be sought, such as private professionals and charities, or even helplines, and it is important to recognize that there is always somewhere you can go, even if it doesn't seem like the most suitable option. At least it is a start.

Once more, this is about your life, your very existence. If you don't fight for you, who will? The key to this is recognizing that if your child, your best friend, your partner or your parent was standing on the edge of a bridge, what would you say? So why won't you say these things to yourself? 'It's hard,' you'll say. 'It's different. It won't stick.' All these things are true, but if you don't stand still and say, 'This is the time when I take responsibility for my life, no matter how hard it is', then who can? Just because it's hard doesn't mean you shouldn't or can't do it. At the end of the day, who cares if you went for therapy? If someone doesn't like it, so what? They aren't feeling awful and living in hell – you are.

You can't rely on pills or on pills alone. The most relevant question to ask yourself is, 'What can I do to help myself?' It's not 'What can pills/doctors/therapists/partners do?' but 'What can I do?' When you start there, you start to take control over your life, and the other things can be added, piece by piece, to help you make your way.

Most people who want to kill themselves don't want to die – they want the feelings to go away but they don't actually want life to end. As you continue reading you'll get to realize that now is not for ever, that how you feel today may be slightly different tomorrow and that life keeps moving, changing, shifting. Suicide is an option but it's not the only option. If you kill yourself then all other options are shutdown, for ever.

If you ask for help, the sky won't fall on your head.

Mindfulness practice: Soles of Your Feet

This is an excellent practice that you can use at any time, such as when you are in a meeting, on a crowded train and starting to feel agitated, if you find your anger creeping in or you are feeling unsure of yourself.

- Place your feet firmly but gently on the ground. Bring your attention to the bottom of your feet, to the soles of your feet.
- Feel the sensation of your foot against your sock, your sock against the bottom of the shoe and your shoe touching the ground. If your feet are bare, then feel the sensation of your bare flesh on the ground.
- Focus all your attention on the soles of your feet.
- In your mind's eye, imagine you are breathing in and out of the soles of your feet.
- Feel each of your feet expanding and then softening with each breath.
- Imagine a sense of weight coming into your feet, and this weight is firm, strong and stabilizing.
- Let this sensation ground you as you breathe in and out.
- Bring your attention back to whatever is happening around you.

Notes to myself

6

No magic pills

How can mindfulness help me?

Mindfulness, combined with psychological concepts and skills, is helpful in the management of anxiety and depression because it involves taking a step back from your thoughts, feelings and reactions and building resilience within yourself. By doing this you can start to engage actively with what leads or contributes to them.

Mindfulness is not relaxation, trying to empty your mind of your anxieties, or a therapy that will cure your depression. Rather it is a way of developing your own internal resources, resilience and balance, which can help you deal with life's challenges and your response to them. It gives you a way of managing your distress so that you feel more in control of it and the events in your life.

Questionnaire

- Do you have worries and thoughts running through your mind, even before you're fully awake?
- Do you have feelings of panic or moments when life seems to be overwhelming?
- Do you have physical symptoms of anxiety or depression, such as palpitations, breathlessness, tiredness, headaches, changes in appetite, disturbed sleep and nausea?
- Do you live with a general feeling of unease and apprehension?

- Do you have little interest in seeing friends and family or doing the things you used to enjoy?
- Do you struggle to imagine a time when you will feel relaxed and happy?
- Do you feel there is no point trying in life as the world always seems to be against you?
- Do you feel as though you've lost hope or feel helpless about your life?

A mindful approach can help you engage with your life and rely on your own abilities to deal with its challenges, rather than looking to an external source of relief such as pills, alcohol, drugs, aggression, sex or work. Research is very active in this field and becoming extensive. It is showing that mindfulness-based interventions have had a number of positive effects, including:

- reducing levels of stress, anxiety and depression;[1,2]
- improving mood and boosting well-being;[3]
- reducing hypertension;[4]
- reducing stress during pregnancy;[5]
- improving the immune system and decreasing painkiller use;[6]
- promoting healthy sleep patterns;[7]
- increasing social[8] and parenting[9] skills;
- improving attention, concentration and motivation at work;[10]
- assisting with addictions[11] and trauma;[12]
- developing coping skills and resilience.[13]

Mindfulness has been shown to be very effective for a range of anxiety and mood disorders, as it helps individuals improve their emotional awareness, responses and resilience.

There are no magic pills

Modern life has led us to believe that there is a quick-fix for every situation. However, this belief does not acknowledge that in many cases, emotional or physical conditions can develop over a long period of time for many different reasons, and there are no pills that can be prescribed to deal with all of them. You didn't wake up one morning and say 'Today I'm going to be depressed' or 'Today I'm going to be overweight.' Weight-loss pills, for example, may promise great things, but without a change in the cause of the problem (for example, the overeating, the psychological reasons behind it, lack of exercise), there will never be any lasting results. Similarly, a quick-fix 'Change your life in five minutes' approach to your anxiety or depression is unlikely to be successful, as there may be a variety of issues to consider if any real shift is to take place. A conscious and thought-through effort is needed on a daily basis.

Like any other skills, mindfulness needs to be nurtured and practised for it to have a positive impact on your life. This requires motivation, openness and a willingness to explore your own life and the choices you make every day, not digging and delving into the deepest parts of your psyche but getting to know the lie of the land within your internal world.

You can't know if someone is an enemy or an ally if you don't know that they exist and you can't know if they'll attack you or support you if you haven't worked out their purpose and aims. The same goes for those different parts of yourself, which is why it is so helpful to have a broader understanding of yourself.

Important

By starting to engage more with your thoughts and by understanding the events that have brought you to where you are now, feelings and memories may be brought to the fore, which could be painful or upsetting. Should this happen, be aware of the sensation but manage it in a positive way, by listening to music or talking to a friend, for example. If the feelings are very distressing you should seek the input of a qualified professional. Therapy should not be regarded as embarrassing or intimidating; it is simply two people coming together to explore your life and develop your understanding of these feelings to deal with them better.

Mindfulness practice: A Moment of Calm in Two Minutes

This two-minute breathing exercise is an excellent introduction to how focusing on your breathing can help to settle and ground you. It's particularly useful when your chest or stomach feels tight, your heart is pounding or you're feeling bombarded by distressing thoughts. It can be done at any time and in any place when you feel off balance or anxious; before giving a presentation or taking an exam, after a difficult conversation, in the staff room at work, even in the bathroom when you just need to take a moment for yourself.

- Sit in a chair with your eyes open or closed and place one hand on your stomach, feeling the rise and fall of it. Without forcing your breath in any way, silently count 'In, two, three, four' on the inbreath and 'Out, two, three, four' on the outbreath. Repeat this three times.

- Breathe in for the same amount of time as above, but count only 'In, two, three' on the inbreath and 'Out, two, three' on the outbreath. Repeat three times, then reduce it to 'In, two', 'Out, two' and repeat three times. Now take one breath in and one breath out, without counting. If this feels difficult, think 'In' and 'Out' to the rhythm of your breathing. Repeat three times.

- Take a moment to think about how you feel. Do you feel calmer? Is your breathing more regular? Do you feel less tense, and have your physical symptoms of anxiety subsided a little? Take away this moment of calm with you, knowing that returning to a calmer and more balanced state of mind can be as simple as breathing.

A note on medication

If you are taking medication and reading this book, you must not stop taking it. If for some reason you think you would like to stop, then you must wait until you have had a discussion with your doctor. Stopping any drug suddenly, including alcohol, is not recommended and should be done gradually in order to prevent side effects, some of which can put you in danger, for example of seizures.

People tend to fall into two categories around the issue of medication. There are those who don't want to go on medication and so they don't tell their doctor how they're feeling. The other set of people are eager to use medication and are either pleased as it's taken the edge off the roller-coaster ride or unhappy as their lives haven't changed very much. In spite of what is said, people frequently stay on medication for an extraordinary number of years without ever having therapy suggested as an alternative or adjunct. People often say that they can't afford therapy. When you recognize that therapy is about your life, for now and the future, then the cost becomes a necessary one. Most people are willing to spend money on a holiday but view therapy as too expensive. It's about recognizing what value you place on your happiness.

Over time there has been an ongoing debate about medication for conditions such as depression and anxiety, especially depression, and there is continuing evidence to suggest that the benefits of therapy are as good as medication.[14,15] The first port of call is usually medication as people tend to go to their doctor for help, but unfortunately, even when there have been only small changes after a period of medication, therapy is rarely suggested as an alternative or even to partner the medication. The main concern here is that people are given the impression that their condition is an illness resulting from a chemical imbalance. There is evidence to suggest that this argument doesn't always apply,[16,17] and one of the dangers is that people don't recognize that they themselves need to work at helping themselves – with or without medication.

There are some individuals who do need medication and it is good that there are suitable types to help them, especially if they are having suicidal thoughts or are highly distressed over a long period. They may, or may not, need to be on it for many years, and if required they must do what is best for them. For others, however, the medication becomes a crutch; the idea of a chemical imbalance corrected by a pill is the answer but perhaps also a way of opting out from standing still and recognizing that they need to deal with their problems and manage their lives. Even if you are one of those people who needs medication for prolonged periods of time, that still doesn't mean you shouldn't be thinking about your struggles, angers and disappointments and finding ways of making sense of them and of developing ways to improve your approach to yourself and to the events and interactions of your life.

Medication is only one treatment, and research shows that mindfulness-based therapy, and other forms of therapy, are as effective as medication.[18] Again, the suggestion is not that you mustn't take medication but that your best way forward, whether or not you take medication, is to build your skills and learn to manage different aspects of your life. When this happens, you then have a fuller understanding of yourself and you have skills that you'll use for the rest of your life in any situation.

Notes to myself

Part 2

How did I get to be like this?

7

Connections

The mind–body connection

The scientific and medical advances of the past few centuries have raised awareness and provided knowledge on what it is to be human. Many diverse fields have emerged, all with different perspectives on the human experience and condition, such as biology, medicine, neuroscience, psychology and anthropology. As a result there has been a move towards dividing the mind and body into separate entities that have minimal interaction. There is an implicit suggestion that humans are composed of a physical 'doing' body, and a non-physical 'thinking, feeling' mind, and that a disorder is either purely physical, such as cancer, or purely mental, such as depression.

Recently, however, there has been better recognition that by reducing the human experience to two separate components we are ignoring the influence the mind can have on the body and vice versa.[1] Think about a time you have been in pain – did it affect your mood, leaving you feeling down or irritable? Now consider a time when your enjoyment of an activity prevented you from realizing you had injured yourself or were in pain. From these examples it can readily be seen that the mind and body interact continually on many different levels, and that understanding the connection between the two can help you manage both physical and emotional conditions.

This mind–body interaction is a beneficial component in understanding conditions, including anxiety and depression, as well as how to manage them. While they may be emotional disorders, both anxiety and depression are often expressed as physical symptoms.[2] Anxiety is known to cause or worsen conditions such as shortness of breath, nausea, headaches, impotence or loss of interest in sex, skin conditions such as psoriasis, palpitations, insomnia or fatigue, restlessness, lethargy and changes in appetite. Depression affects energy levels and sleep patterns, causes loss or gain of weight, reduces interest in sex and is linked to increased alcohol and drug use. It can cause people to be restless, to experience flattened emotion or numbness and to have low self-esteem. It may also cause self-harm or aggressiveness towards others. When considering this range of symptoms, it is clear that anxiety and depression can affect every aspect of your life.

Adopting a mindful approach can help realign the physical and emotional aspects of the self, bringing about balance and well-being that can reduce the symptoms in both mind and body.

The biopsychosocial model

The biopsychosocial model – see Figure 1, opposite – is essentially the concept that your biological, psychological and social make-up interact throughout your life.[3] All three elements are important in forming who you are and how you see the world, and each should be considered within the context of the others and how they interact with and influence each other.

You inherit many of your physical and psychological attributes from your parents through your genes. However, it is your experiences that shape your development. Take for example the process of growing a flower in a pot. All the plant's biological predispositions are contained within the seed that you plant, but its growth and characteristics will also be affected by how often you water it, the quality of the soil, how much sunlight it receives and other factors. In a similar way, humans inherit traits from their parents but their environments and experiences, particularly during early development, lay the

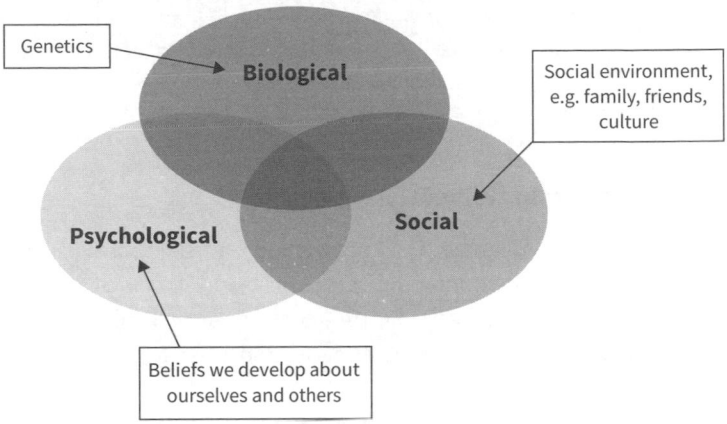

Figure 1 The biopsychosocial model

foundations for their psychological and emotional make-up that will
influence their decisions and choices throughout their lives.

All three elements – biological, psychological and social – contribute to who you are today and have influenced your perception of
the world and your choices, whether consciously or unconsciously.

Take a piece of paper and write down the column headings shown
in Table 1. Using the examples in Figure 1, write in the columns what
you think about yourself and where and why these beliefs may have
come about.

Table 1 Biological, psychological and social influences

Biological	Psychological	Social

When emotions become intensely distressing, you feel the onset of panic or you are overcome by dark thoughts, try taking three deep, conscious breaths. Remind yourself that you have been here before and that the thoughts or feelings will pass.

A note about mindfulness practices

The following practices are designed to help you connect with your body and gain insight into the sensations and tensions you are experiencing. Allow yourself the time and space to really focus on these practices as there is a tendency to find time to invest in our physical health and appearance each day rather than our mental health. Your mind deserves no less attention.

Take a moment to consider your posture as you sit and read this book, walk around the house or go about your daily routine. When you feel distressed or low in mood, you may have a tendency to slump in chairs, move more slowly, look down and have a hunched posture. If you are anxious you may sit on the edge of a chair, move quickly and restlessly, fiddle nervously with objects or be unable to sit still for any length of time. Emotional pain can often affect your posture in the same way as physical pain, leading you to adopt defensive or tense positions. On the other hand, when you are confident and calm, your shoulders will be back, you will stand up straight and look ahead while walking purposefully, or sit comfortably in a chair in an upright, open and relaxed manner. Research has shown that not only do your emotions affect your posture but your posture can also affect your emotions.[4] By adjusting your posture you can lift your mood, reduce aches and pains, improve blood flow around the body and increase your energy levels.

Mindfulness practice: Adjusting Posture

- Sit in a chair in a slumped and hunched position for two minutes. Become aware of your breathing and observe any sensations that come to mind. Can you feel any aches and pains? How is it affecting your breathing? What emotions can you identify?

- Now sit up straighter with your shoulders back. Your posture should be open and relaxed; try to soften your facial muscles and jaw and nurture a feeling of confidence and calm. As you continue to focus on your breathing, notice any changes that occur either physically or emotionally. Do you feel more alert, more confident or less anxious? If no changes occur, that's fine too.

- Make a mental note of your experience and throughout the day become aware of your posture when you feel anxious or distressed. At these times, gently and kindly adjust it if you are hunched, on the edge of your seat or sitting restlessly. Take a moment to think how these small changes may affect your physical and emotional well-being.

Notes to myself

8

The development of self

Getting to be who you are – a psychodynamic approach

Think back to a childhood experience when you were scared, perhaps from getting stuck up a tree or having to tell a parent that you lost your school jumper. Was your fear proportional to the level of risk involved in the situation and the possible consequences? The likelihood is that your level of fear or anxiety was influenced more by your perception of the event than by what actually happened.

A child is only able to understand an experience from the perspective of a child. Even as adults, our perspective on events are coloured by our childhood experiences and interpretation of them. Being an adult doesn't mean that you are now detached or separate from those events and the beliefs and views you took away from them. Frequently it is these early experiences and beliefs that affect how you view both your past and your present life, as well as your future. It is both unrealistic and unhelpful to believe that you can dismiss your past experiences as they have been fundamental influences in shaping who you are today.

While you cannot change your experiences as you were growing up, by going back in your mind and recognizing them and how you interpreted them, you can start to make sense of them and place them within a context. This helps you understand why you attached certain emotions to those experiences and why you interpreted them as you did. Now you can

*reinterpret them as an adult, and some of the older, less helpful beliefs
that came from them. You'll at least have made some sense of them and
be able to intervene when an unhelpful belief starts to play out.*

Start at the beginning

Parents are the most important and influential people in a child's life,
whether they are around or not. From the moment of birth, infants
are able to remember their parents' faces and attach a sense of safety,
security and love to them. If a mother or father – or primary care-
giver – is able to provide the food, warmth, shelter, love, care and
boundaries that a child requires to grow physically and emotionally,
then the child will be able to trust that parent and will develop a
secure attachment to them. This trust provides the blueprint for all
of the child's future relationships, as the child understands that they
are able to trust other people and themselves, allowing them to feel
worthy of love and to love others freely.

If this initial trust and security is not present in their relationship with their parents, then it becomes much harder for children
to believe that they are worthy of love and that others will find them
lovable.[1] At an unconscious level this belief is continued into adult-
hood and may be played out in relationships down the line. Some
people may need constant approval and attention in relationships to
feel valued, or may close themselves off and keep others at a distance
because they do not believe they are loved. These kind of defences
may lead to relationship difficulties that reinforce their belief that
they are unlovable or unworthy, becoming a self-fulfilling prophesy.
These feelings of inadequacy and insecurity can develop into guilt,
shame, distress and anger that then affect people's choices and relationships later in life. As they put defences in place or project these
feelings on to others, their relationships and self-esteem may suffer,
leading to the development of depression or anxiety.[2,3]

Children often believe that an event was caused by their behaviour or personality and are unable to understand the context of the

incident. This can lead to their incorrectly assuming, for example, that their father walked out because they dropped a plate and it smashed, or that their sister became ill because they argued with her. Although this manner of thinking seems illogical to us as adults, it is important to remember that this is how children perceive the world. The emotions that come with these perceptions are very real, affecting them on an unconscious level even as adults. Often for a child it is not the actual event, such as getting lost in a supermarket, that is distressing; rather it is the child's perceptions and beliefs attached to the event, for example, 'Mum forgot about me because she doesn't care about me', that can be disturbing.

Everyone needs protective shields

As a species we are geared at an evolutionary level towards self preservation and survival, so we develop coping strategies and defence mechanisms to help us deal with threatening or difficult experiences.[4] These strategies and defences protect us from anxieties that we fear will overwhelm us, at an unconscious level, and thereby prevent us being engulfed by negative emotions such as fear, sadness or anger.

The difficulty with defences is that they may continue to be in place long after the initial events or emotion have passed, and become part of a general way of dealing with life even though they are no longer needed.

For example, a behaviour that initially was used as a way to manage a situation, such as being quiet to avoid confrontation when a parent has been easily angered, may become generalized to being passive in relationships, being unable to express opinions, leading to frustration and depression. Another example is avoiding peers at school because you have been bullied, which could become generalized to being shy and anxious. From these examples you can see how using this protective shield can remain in place even after the feared situation has passed, eventually becoming a trait or a way of dealing with difficult situations. It is when defence mechanisms interfere with the decisions you make and your relationships with others that they have outlived their purpose and can become disruptive rather than helpful.

At this point it is worthwhile looking back at the events and emotions that activated the mechanism in order to examine the influence it still has on your life. Once you have made sense of how it came about, you can then do something with it as it now has a context into which it can fit.

Take a piece of paper and write down the column headings shown in Table 2. Using the table you previously created (see p. 43) as a foundation, consider some of the factors past and present that could have influenced you and list them in your new table.

Table 2 Factors that have influenced your life

Biological	Psychological	Social	Early experiences	How they affected me

---

Mindfulness practice: The Shower

- While you are in the shower, feel the sensation of the drops of water hitting your skin, the warmth of the water relaxing your muscles and invigorating you.
- Open your mouth, let the drops hit your tongue and feel the water running over your lips and chin.
- Relax into this and become aware of the water against the rest of your body and the sensations that come with that.

Notes to myself

9

Anxiety and depression in context

An anxious mind

Research in neuroscience (the scientific study of the brain and nervous system) has shown that following a traumatic or frightening event, there are physical changes in the brain caused by the release of neurotransmitters (brain chemicals) that mirror psychological reactions.[1] Neuronal (brain) pathways are created that become stronger each time they are activated. This means that when a strategy is activated, such as shouting or withdrawing when someone upsets you, it strengthens the link between the distressing emotion, the psychological reaction and the pathway set up in your brain. This then increases the likelihood that the next time the emotion is experienced, the same reaction will be triggered and the same neuronal pathway activated.[2] Every time you experience that situation or a similar one, your brain immediately puts you on that pathway without you even having to think about it. The pathways are like railway tracks, so if your association puts you on the track going to London, that's the route you'll take even if you want to go to Scotland or cross the seas to New York. The more the pathway is activated the stronger it becomes.

This research shows that not only can we become psychologically conditioned to resort to a certain behaviour or defence mechanism to deal with a distressing emotion, but our brains can also physically change as a result, reinforcing the connection between the emotion and the behaviour. An anxious mind may be predisposed to creating these neuronal pathways more quickly or more deeply, which may account for why anxiety persists long after the event or emotion that triggered it.[3] Some people who suffer from depression may have imbalances in their levels of neurotransmitters, which can affect the way their neuronal pathways work.[4]

The negative bias

Psychologists have established that humans have evolved to have a 'negative bias' in their attention.[5] This means that you attend more to negative events or emotions than to those that are neutral or positive, because they signify potential threats to you. At an evolutionary level you are wired to notice quickly and identify anything that may harm you, allowing you to respond as rapidly as possible.[6] However, this negative bias is also one of the reasons why you sometimes form stronger memories of upsetting experiences than pleasant ones, or tend to focus on the negative aspects of situations. A strong negative bias is one of the underlying reasons behind anxious and depressed thoughts that give rise to feelings of nervousness, apprehension or despair.[7] It can contribute to the feelings of distress and hopelessness experienced by people who have depression or anxiety as it can be difficult to concentrate on the easier or happier moments, and life can look bleak.

Imagine, for example, that you have come home feeling exhausted on a Friday evening after a week at work. As you mentally review your week you remember that your boss was critical of your work or that you have been rushed off your feet all week with no time to relax. Maybe your child was teething and you've had little sleep, you argued with your partner and feel guilty or you developed a cold and the weather was terrible. Perhaps you complain to a family member or partner that you have had a thoroughly bad week, while feeling distressed and tearful. You may want to crawl under the duvet and close yourself off from the world, or you may turn to alcohol to numb your feelings of despair. You could have thoughts that life is not getting any better or that you can't go on living like this.

In this example a negative bias would be contributing to the distressing emotions you feel, as well as colouring your interpretation of your week. Perhaps you have forgotten the laughter you shared with a colleague at lunch, the beautiful sunset you saw on your commute home from work or the unexpected phone call from an old friend. You could have overlooked the moment your favourite song came on the radio and made you smile, or when your partner surprised you with a treat because he or she knew you were having a difficult week. This example illustrates how a negative bias is a key contributing factor to what starts – and then helps to continue – your anxiety and depression. However, it is possible to overcome this type of over-attention to more difficult or distressing aspects of life, through mindfulness practice and recognizing from where the harsh and judgemental views of yourself came.

By practising mindfulness, you will help your brain to gradually develop its executive functions, which include processes such as attention, memory and planning. This reduces the automatic or reactive responses it can give to experiences. In this way, it can shift your perception and understanding of events as your brain has more time to process events and store them once they have had meaning and context put to them.

The most complex organ

A person may be inclined towards anxiety or depression or tend to view things negatively, but this doesn't mean that he or she will develop these disorders. There are predisposing factors in everyone's life towards some anxiety and low mood, yet not everyone suffers from panic attacks or chronic depression. This is because, as already mentioned, the physiology of your brain is not the only aspect contributing to the way you perceive and experience the world. Just as you may have predisposing factors, you also have different aspects that protect you from emotional and mental health issues.[8] These protective factors – such as a good sense of self-worth, a supportive social network, job satisfaction – are as important in understanding your reactions to difficult situations as the anxieties and emotional distress underlying them.

The brain is an extraordinarily complex and fascinating organ as it has the ability to adapt, grow and change according to your experiences. Although neural pathways may be made between distressing emotions and your psychological processes, you can choose to shift your reactions by learning to respond in a different way. Through the mindfulness meditations, you can alter the way you process information and then respond to it. When a neural pathway is activated less, its effect is diminished and the association becomes weaker. Likewise, if you choose to respond to distressing emotions in a more helpful and considered way, new pathways will be created that link the emotions to positive coping mechanisms.[9]

Remember that what fires together wires together, so the more you criticize yourself and focus on the points you dislike, the stronger that pathway becomes. Soften your approach to yourself and you'll not only reduce the strength of those pathways but begin to develop new, more positive ones when you recognize and reinforce a more balanced view of yourself.

There is only one you. Your brain, your mind, your body and your feelings are all interconnected to form who you are right now. All of your experiences, sensations, thoughts and feelings have brought you to where you are today. You cannot change what is in the past but you can choose how to live your life right now, in this moment.

Mindfulness practice: Let's Go for a Walk

This practice is an example of an activity that you do all the time, frequently without paying any attention to what you're doing. It's been adapted from the traditional walking meditation to include a broader perspective. Focusing your attention on your automatic functions can ground and balance you, and this walking practice can be used when anxieties and stresses seem to be getting on top of you. Try it as a short break from work, studying or activities, or when you can feel your frustrations growing.

- Take a walk in the garden, a park or wherever is convenient. Keeping your eyes lowered, bring your attention to the physical sensations of walking. Feel the changes in pressure as you place your feet on the ground, be aware of your breathing, pay attention to the rhythm of your footsteps and the slight swinging motion of your arms. Acknowledge any emotions or sensations that come into your mind.

- Lift your eyes to the world around you. Little by little pay special attention to the sights, sounds and smells of your environment. Take everything in: the movement, the stillness, the light, the shade, the chaos and the peace. Allow yourself to be open to your environment and its effect on you.

- Shift your focus to your connection to the outside world and the impact you are having on your environment. Let your breathing flow naturally, becoming part of the world around you. Feel the stability of the ground beneath your feet and let it strengthen you. Notice any changes in the sensations and feelings you are experiencing and acknowledge that the world around you is having an impact on you, just as you have an influence on the environment.

- Finally, take a mental step back from such an active involvement in the sensations of the environment. Continue to observe your breathing gently as a space forms between you and the outside world. You are aware of your surroundings, sensitive to them and appreciative of them, but the sensations arising from them are not the entirety of your experience. Take a moment to appreciate this moment, knowing you can take this sense of peace and clarity with you when you step back into your everyday activities.

Notes to myself

10

The stress response

Understanding stress

So far there has been discussion around the broad picture of your brain and how certain aspects might make you more prone to depression or anxiety. But it is just as important to look at the processes occurring in your nervous system in the short term, to learn how stress affects your body and how to manage feelings of stress, anxiety or depression on a daily basis.

The only moment in time that you can truly know and understand is now. Whatever has gone before is in the past and you cannot know what the future will be. Shifting your focus to the present allows you to be aware and to bring balance to your life from this moment to the next one.

Stress affects your body at a physical level just as much as it affects you emotionally, whether you notice it or not. When your brain senses fear or danger it shifts into its survival mode. This is because you have evolved to display the fight or flight response when you are threatened, which prepares your body either to defend you or run away.[1] Unfortunately the primal parts of your brain that activate this response cannot tell the difference between stress caused by physical threats, such as a sabretooth tiger trying to eat you, and psychological threats to your well-being, such as the printer breaking down, or feeling rejected by a loved one. So in either case your body would prepare the fight or flight response, and the processes underlying the response are triggered.

There is also a possible third response in this scenario, which is freezing in the style of a rabbit-in-the-headlights. This option occurs when overwhelmed by fear, which causes you to be physically or psychologically immobilized or else retreat into yourself.[2] This can occur when you have found that the safest option in threatening situations has been not to react, and is common when someone has been abused or exposed to ongoing threats to their well-being.

Punching the sabretooth tiger

When the fight or flight response is activated, your brain kicks your body into gear by activating the sympathetic system of your autonomic nervous system. Stress hormones, such as adrenaline and cortisol, get released and start shutting down all the systems you don't need. This is similar to the way a computer shuts down all other programs when installing updates; all of the parts of the body that are not essential for your impending escape or death-defying struggle are temporarily put on the back burner. In the case that you were in fact about to be the sabretooth tiger's lunch, this would allow all of your energy to be poured into making you run faster or punch the tiger harder. Your heart would beat faster, pumping more oxygen around the body, and blood would rush to your muscles, filling them with the energy you may need to increase your chances of survival.

The extra energy being used in your muscles in this scenario would be redirected from your digestive system and the not-unimportant tasks of digestion, absorption and excretion. This means that your body is unable to replenish the energy it is expending while fighting the tiger. In addition, the stress hormones that are released can have negative effects on the body, causing important functions such as your immune system to suffer. This is because the stress hormone corticosteroid lowers the amount of lymphocytes in your bloodstream, which are a type of white blood cell responsible for killing dangerous cells, such as infections, viruses and tumour cells.[3] The stress response therefore leaves you lacking energy, less able to repair damaged tissues and more vulnerable to the effects of harmful bacteria and viruses.[4]

After the struggle

Once the threat has gone (you have defeated the tiger, climbed a tree to hide or (in the case of an everyday cause of stress) the traffic has started to move), your body has to return to its original state. The parasympathetic system kicks in, reducing your high-alert state and working to restore your bodily functions to normal. Exhaustion or tiredness kicks in while your body tries to catch up on the digestive and immune functions that were dampened down during the fight or flight response (see Figure 2).

However, in the modern world the fight or flight response is not so simple. While you might not have to battle sabretooth tigers, you are exposed to psychological threats and stressors all the time and rarely have the time to relax fully to recoup your energy. Life can sometimes feel like a constant battle, and the stress response can become overactivated (see Figure 3, opposite). This can lead to stress hormones such as adrenaline and cortisol being released when they

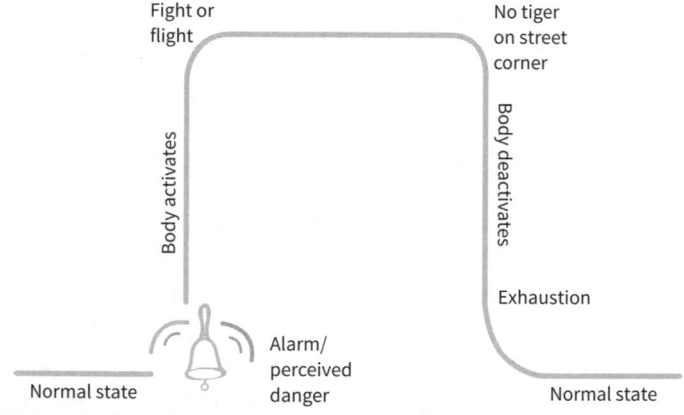

Figure 2 The stress response

are not needed, causing physical symptoms of stress such as heart palpitations and breathlessness.[5] Nausea and stomach aches can be caused by the effect of the digestive system being dampened down, energy levels decrease causing lethargy, and if the stress response is sustained over a long time, the immune system can suffer (leading to increased illness and susceptibility to infection), fat deposits accumulate around your middle (putting you at greater risk of heart disease) and your organs begin to be worn down.[6] In addition, when stress becomes a chronic problem, the body becomes confused and releases either too much or too little of the stress hormones, causing problems with the regulation of the sympathetic nervous system.[7]

It's easy to see how these effects can cause you to become physically and psychologically exhausted. Now bear in mind that people with anxiety or depression may have an overly sensitive stress response system,[8] and it becomes apparent that anxiety, stress and depression can have not only lasting psychological effects but also pose a threat to your overall physical and mental health. Learning to intervene before the stress response kicks in can help to reduce the negative effects of anxiety and depression, decreasing physical symptoms and promoting a sense of balance and well-being.

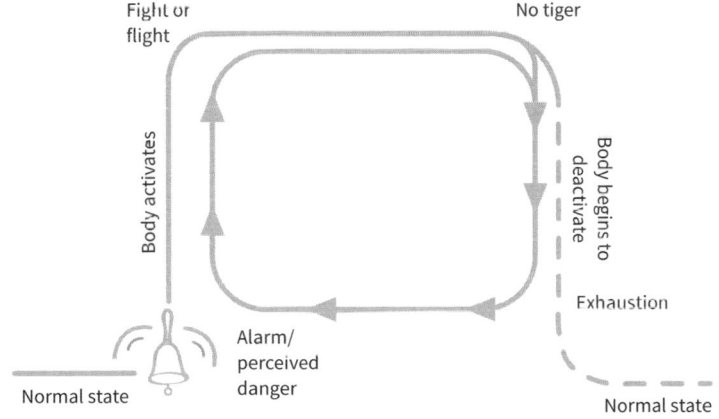

Figure 3 The chronic/ongoing stress response

Mindfulness practice: Body Focus

Find a quiet place to carry out this practice. Switch your phone to silent or leave it in another room; ask others around you not to disturb you unless it's an emergency. Ensure you are wearing comfortable clothing and that you will be warm enough; perhaps have a blanket nearby, as your body temperature will drop. This is also an excellent practice for dealing with physical pain.

- Choose a position that is comfortable and works well for you. The ideal position is lying flat on your back on the floor (Figure 4), on a rug or blanket if there is no carpet, with a cushion for your head if this increases your comfort.

- Place your legs on a chair, straight or bent, if that is easier on your back (Figure 5). An alternative is lying on a bed, especially if you have difficulty getting to the floor; perhaps complete this practice early in the day if you are using a bed however, to help avoid falling asleep. If lying down is uncomfortable or difficult for you, you can sit in a chair that provides

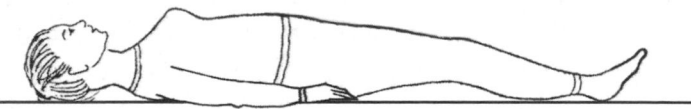

Figure 4 Lying on the floor

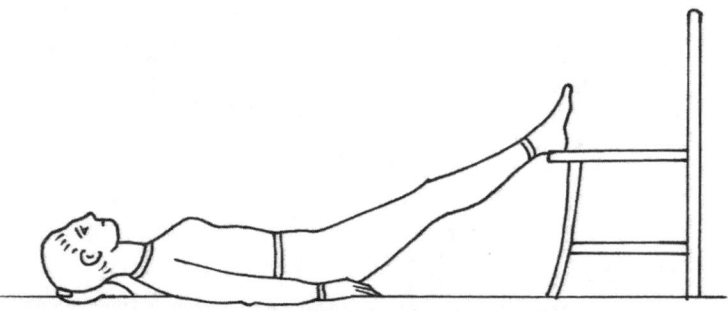

Figure 5 Lying on the floor with feet up on a chair

sufficient support (Figure 6, overleaf), using footstools or cushions to ensure your comfort. If sitting is not ideal you can stand or lean against a wall, ensuring you have a steady object to lean on (Figure 7, overleaf).

- A note about breathing: When the audio download says 'breathe into your toes' or any other part of your body, it is meant metaphorically. Physiologically we are unable to breathe into any part of our body other than our lungs, so it is about imagining the breath moving through your body. By placing your breath into an area of your body in your imagination, you are bringing attention and focus to it and relaxing the area.

- Before starting the practice, take a moment to think about how you are feeling. Take note of any physical sensations of stress or anxiety, as well as any thoughts or emotions that are at the forefront of your mind. Tell yourself that this is very important for your psychological and physical well-being.

🔊 Listen to the Body Focus practice, which you will find in the audio downloads that go with this book. A written sample of the wording of the practice can be found below. It has been included so that you can get an idea of what it is about and be reassured that there is nothing in any of the practices that aims to put you into a trance-like or altered state of mind. All you are doing is breathing.

After the practice, take a few moments to think about your response to it before moving. Did you give yourself the time and space to do the practice? What were your expectations before the practice, and were they reasonable? For example, did you expect to feel much calmer but now feel frustrated because you still feel stressed? Were you cynical at first, but found the practice enjoyable and relaxing?

Most people fall asleep when they first do this practice. However, if you find that you continually fall asleep when doing it then it is helpful to do it sitting up until you are able to remain alert throughout. The purpose of the practice is to bring awareness to your body, not send you off to sleep.

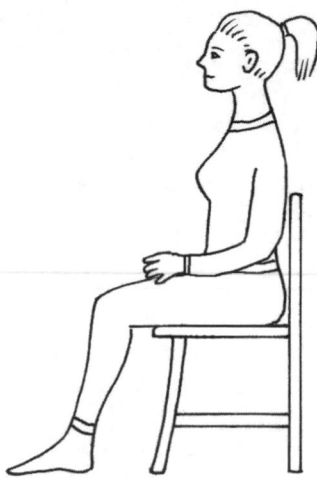

Figure 6 Sitting in a chair

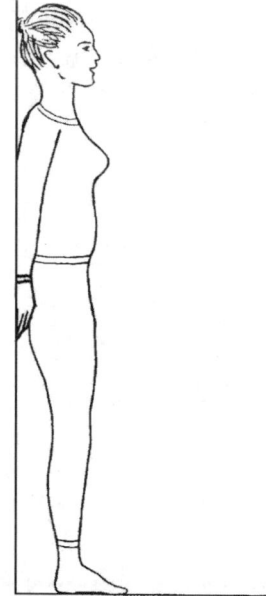

Figure 7 Standing against a wall

Extract from the transcript of the Body Focus practice

The intention is to bring awareness to the different parts of the body without moving or stretching them in any way. It is about experiencing the sensations within your body, making no demands on it.

As you breathe in and out, become aware that this is your body, all of it, for whatever it is: the parts that work well and keep you alive as well as the parts that are damaged and in pain.

Now focus on the big toe of your left foot. Become aware of the existence of this part of your body and the sensations that might be there. Let your attention go deep into the toe – not moving it, just observing it and feeling whatever is or isn't happening in it at this moment. If you feel no sensations, that too is fine. Simply acknowledge whatever is there.

Now move your focus to the little toe on the left foot – and to all the toes. Become aware of the feelings within the toes, acknowledge them, and breathe deep into the toes on an inbreath. And on an outbreath, let go of your awareness of the toes, letting their existence drift and dissolve from your mind.

Now bring your attention to the sole of your left foot, focusing on any sensations deep within the foot, aware of the air against it, your instep, the heel against the floor. Breathe in and out of it, and on the outbreath, let go of your awareness of it and bring it to the top of the left foot, becoming familiar with the sensations in this part of your body, of all the small bones that make up the foot. Breathe all the way into it and then on an outbreath, let it dissolve from awareness.

Move your focus to the left ankle, feeling and acknowledging whatever it is that's there, aware of the bones that come together to form a joint. Breathe into it and out of it, letting it go. Now focus on the foot and ankle as a whole, breathing deep into it. Let your breath travel, in your mind's eye, all the way down from the nostrils, through the chest and abdomen, down the left leg and into the foot and ankle, aware of the oxygen coming to it. And when it gets there, release and let the breath travel all the way back out through the nostrils, and on an outbreath, let the foot and ankle dissolve from your awareness.

Remember, the practices are there to help you to switch on, not to switch off.

Notes to myself

Part 3

Breaking the cycle

11

Effects of mindfulness on the brain

Intercepting the stress response

Mindfulness has been shown to have a positive effect on the brain because the practices and approach can intercept the stress response before it has damaging effects from unnecessary activation.[1] That is not to say that by practising mindfulness you will never be anxious or depressed. Rather, by developing a mindful approach to life you will be able to deal with distressing or fearful situations as they arise, avoiding the chronic exposure to stress hormones that can cause the physical problems and mental exhaustion previously discussed. In addition, mindfulness may help to regulate release of neurotransmitters and increase the number of connections between different areas of the brain.[2] These physical changes in the brain then give rise to improved function, which can influence your emotional state.

The evidence

New brain-imaging technologies have enabled psychologists and neuroscientists to study the effects of mindfulness in new and advanced ways. Functional magnetic resonance imaging (fMRI) scans are able to give precise visual indications of changes in brain structure before and after adopting mindfulness practices, as well as comparing the brains of people who practise mindfulness and those who don't.

The research shows that mindfulness meditation can:

- increase the brain's grey matter in areas responsible for regulating emotions, sensations and thoughts;[3]
- increase impulse control[4] and improve reasoning and decision-making skills;[5]
- improve executive functions such as memory and attention;[6]
- decrease stress and levels of stress hormones, improve quality of life, improve mood, decrease levels of depression and reduce the effects of trauma;[7]
- improve quality of sleep, promote a sense of happiness and improve relationship satisfaction.[8]

Mindfulness has therefore been proven to be effective for many of the issues facing people who have anxiety or depression.

The importance of breathing

Much of the effectiveness of mindfulness can be traced back to its emphasis on the most basic of functions: breathing. Breathing is essential for survival, but it also plays a key role in the management of stress. If you have ever been comforted while you were nervous, panicking or sobbing and inconsolable, it is likely that you have been told to 'take deep breaths' to calm down. Although everyone instinctively knows how to breathe, we do not necessarily know how to breathe well. We have a tendency to breathe into the shallowest part of our lungs, which have the least flexibility and space. The effect of this is that the amount of air entering our lungs is reduced and the pattern of our breathing is shallow and irregular.

If you have watched a child or partner sleeping, recall how peaceful they looked as their chest rose and fell in a rhythmic way, their shoulders relaxed and their breathing came easily and naturally in a deep, smooth and calming rhythm. Now consider your breathing at this moment in time. Is it similar to that deep, calm and natural rhythm or is it shallow and irregular? Does your breath feel shaky or fast-paced? Is your chest tight?

Although breathing is a natural and automatic process, by paying attention to it you will find that you may not be breathing as effectively as you could be. By noticing your breathing and focusing on it during the practices and at other times, you can increase the levels of oxygen entering your bloodstream and your brain, reduce your stress levels and the release of stress hormones, as well as promote your own sense of well-being. You will also be building your internal resilience and resourcefulness, and gaining more awareness of why you respond as you do and how you can have control over your reactions and responses to what you feel, think and do and the choices that you make.

Meditation or sitting positions

The meditation positions, or sitting positions as they are often called, are illustrated in Figures 4–7 in Chapter 10. You may find it more comfortable sitting upright in a chair, on your bed or cross-legged on the sofa. Some people find it very focusing to sit on a meditation cushion. These are often large, firm, round cushions called zafus, which help you to keep upright. It is important whenever you are sitting for any period of time to make sure that the level of your hips is higher than your knees, even when sitting in a chair. There is no need for you to suffer, so use props, cushions, blankets or anything else to help you feel comfortable, but always try to keep your back upright, your chest and heart area open and your head gently balanced on your neck. There should be a softness and openness to your approach to all the practices. There will always be noise, but try to find a place where you won't be interrupted, and ensure that your mobile phone is turned down. These meditations can be done whether sitting at an office desk, in a chair at home or on a bench in the garden.

No right or wrong way

When doing these practices there is no set way or special position. What helps is knowing that your mind will drift whenever you do a practice and that your thoughts will suddenly take on great importance now that you're trying to let them pass on and are not sticking with each one. Minds drift and float, they think and produce pictures, thoughts, ideas, sensations and many other things – and that's because they are doing exactly what they're meant to do. Trying to stop this happening is pointless. What you want is to start to be aware of how these thoughts come to mind, what they are and how you can manage them. Acknowledge whatever is there without reacting, simply saying 'Thought' when a thought comes up or 'Feeling' when a feeling emerges. It's about recognizing the activity for what it is – for example, thinking – and then letting it be there without attending to it.

When your concentration moves from your breathing or when you find yourself getting into a conversation with yourself, or someone else in your head, about a topic, recognize this activity, step away from it and bring your attention back to your breathing – focus and refocus no matter how often this happens. This will happen repeatedly – for years to come – because your mind and brain are doing what they're meant to do. Your task is to manage your thoughts and responses, and it is this management of them that will help to make such a difference to your life. Training yourself to recognize, acknowledge and let pass difficult, repetitive and unwarranted thoughts, self-criticism and judgement will not only provide relief but reset your attitude and brain pathways so that you can open up your life to kindness and balance. You won't need to go down each dark alley in your mind because, with practice, you'll be able to stop, recognize what you're doing and reset your path on to something far more helpful and nourishing.

It cannot be stressed enough how essential it is that you keep doing the practices as each time you do, you're developing the structures in your brain, your emotional resilience and your own internal sense of stability and belief.

Mindful awareness

The following practice is one that you will come to rely on for years to come. It is one of the key meditations that is central to mindfulness practice, and its benefits are far reaching. It truly is worth doing on a regular basis, even if only for five or ten minutes a day.

Mindfulness practice: Mindful Awareness

Mindful awareness is about becoming aware of what is happening within yourself, which encourages you to bring your focus and attention to your internal experiences and how they shift.

🔊 There are two options for this practice on the audio download: a 20-minute and a 5-minute version. Begin with the 5-minute version, and once this feels familiar you can then move on to the 20 minute one if you can. Ideally, do the 20-minute version a few times per week and the 5-minute one on the other days.

Below you will see a transcript of the 5-minute Mindful Awareness practice, which is a breathing practice. It has been included to show you that there is nothing strange or peculiar about the practices. You are breathing anyway, so these practices help you to focus your breathing and to use it in a remarkably helpful way.

Transcript of the Mindful Awareness practice (5-minute version)

With your eyes closed, while being alert and awake, bring your attention to your breathing and to the movement of the breath as it comes in and out of your body. Simply observe your breathing – watching the path it takes as it travels in at the nose, down to the abdomen and then out again through the nose.

Stay focused on the breath, without forcing it in any way. Be here, with each inbreath and with each outbreath, letting one follow on from the other.

Use your breath as an anchor. Allow the breath to anchor you to the centre within your abdomen, that part that is stable, focused and present. Follow the breath to your anchor, bringing with it a new beginning and with each outbreath a letting go.

Be aware of each breath nourishing and grounding you, renewing and letting go, one breath following the other. Allow it to bring with it a stillness and a feeling of balance, grounding you right here, right now. Letting it anchor you, gently and kindly, to this moment, and to this moment.

As the intensity begins to ease, let your attention spread to include all of your body, and engage your breath into a rhythmic flow that moves in and out of your body as a whole.

Gradually let your awareness begin to take in the sounds around you and within you, simply letting them exist in harmony with you, as you breathe. Sit in stillness, in this moment.

Feel grounded, feel balanced. Gently allow all of your senses to be awake, to be alert and alive to all that is happening within you and around you. Acknowledge with kindness that you spent this time living each moment of your life, with whatever came with it, in a mindful, balanced and open way, and that you now have the choice of how you wish to live this moment of your life, and this moment.

A moment of thought

After a few weeks of doing the practices, think about what it was like when you first started doing them or even back to the time before you started. Have you made the effort or do you skip over the practices and only read them or about them?

Make a mental note or use your 'Notes to myself' to see if you have noticed any positive or negative effects of the practices. Do you feel that you have been managing stressful situations differently since you have started exploring mindfulness work? What has motivated you to continue?

If you have been doing the practices, what made you do them and how do you keep them going?

If you haven't, think about why not. You may find that there are similarities between this and how you generally approach new or difficult things in your life. Now is the time for you to either use the motivation that you have to keep going or address the lack of interest or procrastination that has prevented you from moving forward.

This is a key issue as it underlies how you interpret and engage with what is offered to you as something that can help, and how you then use these offerings in any meaningful way.

The idea behind the approach in this book is to help you develop awareness of yourself and to encourage you to increase your own sense of resilience and belief that you are the one person who can make the most difference in your life.

Notes to myself

12

A vicious cycle

History repeating itself

Have you ever felt that history seems to be repeating itself and that you continue to make the same mistakes or end up in the same situations again and again? People have a tendency to repeat patterns for several reasons. First, a pattern of behaviour, thoughts or emotions may be repeated even though you know or expect the outcome to be distressing, because it is familiar. Change is difficult and evokes a lot of anxiety, so often it is easier to follow a path that leads to an upsetting but familiar outcome than one that will lead to unknown consequences.

You may choose painful or distressing routes at an unconscious level, which is why it is important to understand what drives you to make these choices.

An example of this type of repetition is someone who has low self esteem and likes to feel needed in a relationship. The person may then choose unsuitable partners who are happy to be dependent on them and end up taking advantage of them. Although this pattern always leads to the same conclusion, such as unhappiness and the break up of the relationship, it is easier to deal with than the uncertainty that could come from a relationship that has a different dynamic.

The second reason that people tend to repeat patterns of behaviours is because they hope that this time the outcome will be different. Perhaps there have been times when you have thought 'Maybe this time John will treat me better' or 'Maybe this time things will sort themselves out', but the outcome has been the same as before.

Ideas perpetuated in books, magazines, films and television suggest that if you want something enough, or have enough hope, you will get your wish. However, this is rarely the case, as wanting or hoping for something, or imagining that you are drawing it towards you, is not the same as working hard and putting in the effort to make a real change. Hope is not helpful unless it is accompanied by motivation and determination. There is no substitute for doing the right sort of work and having a willingness to keep on trying to make things different. Shifting old patterns and managing new and old experiences takes commitment. Just as you brush your teeth twice a day to keep your gums and mouth healthy, so you need to do the same with your mental and psychological health.

The transience of life

When you feel stuck in a cycle that keeps repeating itself or you feel as if life is not getting any better, you can become fixed on either the events that happened to you in the past or on your projections of what the future will bring. The difficulty with this approach is that you plant yourself firmly in a time that is impossible to experience truly or understand, reliving painful memories or becoming anxious about what is to come. At this time it can be helpful to remember one of the fundamental ideas of mindfulness, which is that the most important time is the present.

Life is transient, and moments of both despair and happiness naturally shift as time moves on. Learning to move with time rather than struggling against it is a helpful part of this work.

By now you should have experienced at least one of the mindfulness practices, perhaps the Body Focus or Mindful Awareness practice (see pages 62 and 73). There were probably times when there was a sensation (an itchy foot) or emotion (feeling frustrated) that came up and then drifted off almost unnoticed. At another time, when you may have felt a growing sense of unease or a sudden shot of sadness, recall if it lessened naturally with time.

Fighting against an emotion increases its intensity and its impact on your life. Next time you have a wave of difficult feelings, try breathing into it, knowing that each inbreath can dissipate its force and grip. Bring to mind as you breathe that you can let it out and lessen its intensity. Each breath is a new beginning. That may sound silly, but when you recognize that each moment of your life is a new moment and that the one that has just passed can never be again, it makes more sense.

The Buddhists talk of 'beginner's mind', which denotes bringing to each new or old experience an attitude as though it is happening for the first time. You can try it in all situations, but easy ways are when eating a meal, walking to the shop, taking a bath or having sex with an established partner.

Just like the breath, thoughts and emotions come and go. When you sit quietly and observe them you can notice their impermanence and their intensity may start to fade.

Mindfulness practice: The Mountain Meditation

The Mountain Meditation is designed to create a sense of stability, balance and well-being. It is about claiming this moment and this space for yourself, and anchoring yourself to the present moment no matter how difficult or distressing life may be. The Mountain Meditation is a reminder of inner resilience, reassuring you that you can weather any storm.

◀)) Listen to the Mountain Meditation audio download. Afterwards, take a few moments to reflect on how you face difficulties. Think about the storms you have weathered, the times you thought you couldn't cope or that life was not going to get better. Hold in your mind what you think helped you get through it.

No matter how chaotic and unkind life may seem at times, you have the ability to develop and encourage that strength within you. Even at times when you feel you are weak, that you are failing or when you believe you can't face life's challenges, there is a strength within you that you can draw on to help you manage the pain, fear, distress and despair that life can inflict.

Whenever your anxieties or depression become distressing or harsh, know that you can return to this stable and resilient place. Thoughts, feelings, emotions and experience are transient, but the core of you is constant and enduring. By practising such exercises as The Mountain and Mindful Awareness, you are developing your own ability to manage your difficult emotions, reinforcing your ability to make a choice of well-being over anxiety or happiness over distress. Mindfulness is as much about celebrating your achievements, your success, your health and your well-being as about overcoming the more negative experiences and aspects of your life.

Transcript of the Mountain Meditation

Stand with your feet hip-width apart so that you can balance yourself. Keep your knees soft and your hips loose, imagining there is a small weight attached to your tailbone (coccyx). Tuck your navel in towards your spine as though you are pulling in your stomach to tighten your belt. Relax your shoulders into your back, lightly tuck in your chin and let your head balance on top of your spine. Breathe in, and on an outbreath let unwanted tension be released. On an inbreath take in a feeling of relaxed strength.

As you stand, be aware of your breath moving in at the nostrils, down the back of the throat, into the chest and down into the abdomen, and then of its movement from the abdomen, through the chest and throat and out through the nose. Allow a natural rhythm of breathing, not forcing the breath in or out in any way.

While standing here, feel the weight of your body in your feet, firm against the earth, and that the earth can carry your weight with confidence. Let your breath feel as if it is moving all the way down into your feet, giving them strength and stability. Now let the breath move into your ankles, strengthening them, and now into the calves. Let it flow into your knees, without locking them, and then into your thighs. Move the breath and steadiness into your hips, genitals, buttocks and abdomen, and let this area of your body feel strong but relaxed.

Allow the breath and strength to move up your spine at the back, through your stomach and chest, eventually reaching your shoulders, checking that they are relaxed. Your arms become stronger and part of the mountain, stabilizing you, balancing you. Let the breath move into your neck and jaw, into the skull, ears, face, eyes and right up to the top of your head.

Now, in your mind's eye, move the breath to the base of your spine and thread it like a piece of string through each vertebra from the tailbone, up through the pelvis, the lower back, the middle of your back, the shoulder-blade area, the back of the neck and all the way to the top of your head, where it exits and is held gently but firmly on a hook, allowing your body to hold itself.

Feel the sensation of this, of your body standing like a mountain, fixed and firm, gracious and solid. The mountain is stable and grand: the earth beneath it, the sky and air around it. The weather changes, the seasons move from one to another but the mountain remains. Feel the strength of the earth beneath you, solid and powerful, and your body open and alert, as you stand grounded and dignified in this space.

Notes to myself

13

Why me?

Reasons, not excuses

At times you may be quick to criticize and be hard on yourself for what you think and how you behave, or even for your perceived deficiencies, when you wouldn't inflict judgement on others in the same way. It helps to remember that understanding the reasons behind your behaviour is not the same as making excuses for it. It can feel uneasy or distressing to take a closer look at your anxieties or what has lead to your feeling and staying depressed, as it can seem like admitting failure or defeat: 'I have a nice house, a wonderful family, a stable job. What have I got to be depressed about? It is selfish and ungrateful of me to be unhappy. I have no right to feel angry because that would seem disloyal to someone who loves me.'

You may feel that you should be strong and battle on through life's difficulties, feeling guilty for not being happy or fully appreciative of what you have. Alternatively, you may be confused and at a loss as to why you feel as you do. Most likely you'll be harsh on yourself for being so useless and for not pulling yourself together and getting on with it.

There is no shame in feelings. Mindfulness, within the context of this book, is about taking the time to bring a gentle focus to the different aspects of yourself and see them with kindness rather than with criticism.

It helps to create a more open and accepting, even honest, relationship with yourself and to place your life and these feelings into context. This will allow you to understand better where your feelings are coming from and develop a kind and nurturing attitude towards yourself. No one can thrive on criticism and negativity, and it is exhausting when you're battling yourself as well as all of life's struggles.

Avoiding thoughts

When you actively try to avoid thoughts that make you uncomfortable or distressed you can end up making them more intense.[1] When you actively try to shut out painful or fearful thoughts and feelings you are activating the neural pathways more, causing the thoughts and associations to occur more often. When you are depressed or anxious, thoughts may occur that are shocking or distressing to you: you may fantasize of harming yourself or someone else, have judgemental or spiteful thoughts about others or have repetitive thoughts about how you feel life should be or what you should have done differently. It is important to remember that thoughts do not exist outside of the mind (your mind), and have no bearing on reality (your mind, your thoughts). If you feel guilt, shame or distress because of your thoughts, you can refocus your energies not on avoiding them but on facing them. Mindfully accepting the thoughts with openness and curiosity is one way to remind yourself that you don't need to attach to these thoughts; they will come and go and you can choose whether or not to believe them or focus on them. By redirecting energy from avoidance to acceptance you can start to observe your thoughts in a more detached way, learning to recognize where they come from and which emotions accompany them. This knowledge can take the power out of the thought, relaxing its grip on your mind and reducing the likelihood of it recurring.

The one aspect of your thoughts that you shouldn't ignore or step away from are any thoughts that involve you actually harming yourself or someone else. These thoughts and ideas need to be looked at, and you really should seek help if they are present in your mind in any significant way, particularly if you are making any form of plans around them, even in a detached way.

Thoughts only have power if you give them power, especially if you fear them so much that you push them away or suppress them. By inviting dark thoughts into the light in a manner of acceptance and curiosity, you can learn to choose which thoughts to believe and which to accept as nothing more than a story.

Mindfulness is not about stopping or changing your thoughts but about forming a different relationship with them.

Finding the balance

Criticism and censure can be unhelpful when experiencing difficulties in life and it is far more helpful to maintain a balanced view of your life to ensure that anxiety or depression does not define who you are. During hard times it is easy to lose perspective on who you are and your abilities. At times, self-pity or an overdependence on others for reassurance can creep in. For example, you may think or say that it's your partner's fault you're depressed or that your boss is to blame; you may be angry with life for not being nicer to you, or think that it's unfair that some people have all the luck. Such thoughts aren't uncommon, even if they aren't expressed to others, but they can also lead you to start feeling helplessness, which will add to your state of distress and can therefore deepen depression or exacerbate anxiety.

Mindfulness practice: Choosing to Refocus

If you notice thoughts of pity or helplessness occurring, take a moment to take a few careful breaths, anchoring yourself to the present while you observe the thoughts. Recognize that they are thoughts, your thoughts but only thoughts, stories your mind has told you that you don't have to believe or hold on to. Remind yourself that you don't need to attach any significance to the thoughts. With curiosity and openness, sit quietly with any emotions associated with the thoughts. Now shift your attention on to an aspect of your present experience that feels kinder or easier; perhaps the warmth of the sunshine on your skin or the soft rug on the soles of your feet. No matter how small or insignificant, sit with the experience and appreciate the moment for what it is. Choosing to refocus your attention is a step towards taking responsibility for your life and developing emotional resilience.

Notes to myself

Part 4

Working with, not against, yourself

14

Firefighting anxieties and depression

Life is hard

Life can often feel like repeatedly being buffeted from one crisis to another, reacting to situations as they occur without having the time or energy to stop and consider where you're going or what you're trying to achieve. Being stuck on a hamster-wheel running at a faster and faster pace without end is something most people can identify with.

Taking time to consider your life in a thoughtful and mindful way can give you the mental space and perspective you need to think about the choices you make and their effect on your life.

By learning to focus your attention and getting to know yourself, you can start to ask the questions that will help you to move forward.

- Why do I do this? What are my motivations? Am I making an active choice, or is this behaviour my typical reaction to the situation?
- Have I been here before? – Does this situation, relationship or way of thinking seem familiar?
- What happened last time I chose this route? – What can I expect if I repeat my actions? Is that the outcome I want?
- Where do I want to go? – Am I simply trying to get back to a place

that I know is familiar, or do I want to look at doing something in a different way? What is holding me back?

Fighting fires

These types of questions can be difficult to think about as there is a tendency to push aside the big issues in order to fire fight the seemingly endless annoyances and anxieties of everyday life.

Developing a mindful mindset can help shift the focus from constantly fighting fires in a frantic way to understanding what fuels them and how some may be prevented. It's about taking care of yourself by putting the alarms in place. That way, a small flame can be dealt with before it becomes an all-consuming inferno.

You may feel that things in your life are beyond your control or that you are powerless to change aspects of your life. Feelings of anxiety, fear or panic can become overwhelming and it can be difficult to see how things can be different. By stepping back, focusing on your breathing and building your resilience, you can learn to make choices in a thoughtful and considered manner rather than as a panicked reaction, and bring about a sense of control and ease in your life.

Knowing your options

You may not necessarily believe it, but you do have a choice – although it will take time and ongoing work to make it a reality. Depression and anxiety can stop you enjoying things you did in the past, lose friendships, reduce the number of social events you attend (even if you really do want to be there), and many other things. They can also affect your personal relationships with your partner, your children, your close friends, and be a barrier to engaging with them and enjoying the time you spend together. You may even try to avoid being with them in any meaningful way, or avoid them in other ways, such as in solitary pursuits or watching television, in order to avoid conversation and the like. Drumming up the enthusiasm to go out and participate may make you feel nervous, self-conscious or exhausted before you've even left the house. Getting to know what lies behind your feelings and situation and developing mindfulness can help generate motivation and interest in your life, which will expand your options and increase your sense of balance and enjoyment. There's no point carrying a heavy, disabling rucksack around with you all day if you don't know why you're doing it or what's in it. It is by putting the rucksack down, seeing the rocks inside it and recognizing each for what it is that you can then do something about the situation. Things seldom get better on their own.

Give this a try

Take a piece of paper and a pen and divide the page into two. On one side, write down any interests you have had in the past; it can be anything from horse-riding lessons as a child to attending dance classes with a colleague or even visiting the local pub. On the other side of the page, write down any activities or interests you would like to try or would participate in if things were different or you had more time; this may be as adventurous as paragliding or as simple as baking a cake. Keep this piece of paper as a reminder of the options you have for expanding your life and interests, and use it as motivation to try something new.

Notes to myself

15

Moving forward

One breath at a time

Life is about moving forward, one breath at a time. By focusing on the present moment you can acknowledge and move from the past, knowing that while you cannot change past experiences, you can change the way they affect your life, now and in the future. You can begin to gently quieten your anxieties and distress, knowing that there is a strength and resilience to cope. And if you feel you don't have the strength, then know that you can develop it by building on the skills you already do have. Everyone has some skills and resources, otherwise they wouldn't be able to survive. Letting go of your fears, hurts and angers is a daunting prospect, but you don't need to let go of them, you need to learn to manage them in a different way so that your life isn't being held back.

By looking at past experiences and becoming aware of some of the events and emotions that brought you to where you are today, it is possible to start to release the intensity of the grip of these painful feelings.

Pleased to meet you

You may be feeling that you are defined by the problems you've been struggling with, but that is not true. You are still you for all of your feelings, and each part of you needs to learn to co-exist with the other parts, to live together without denying or trying to avoid

95

one set of parts in favour of others. You can gradually develop your ability to care about all of yourself, as you are now, and to appreciate your present moment for all that you are, even if you view some of it as flawed.

Mindfulness can provide a way to come home to yourself, to get to know yourself in a different way.

Depression and anxiety can shine a spotlight on your weaknesses, fragility, shame and guilt. During these times it's difficult to see how you can move forwards, and it can start to feel as if you're not deserving of happiness. You become your own worst enemy, your harshest critic and your least loved person. However, everyone has the chance to make choices every day about their lives, and the responsibility for your life is in your hands. Everyone deserves happiness and well-being, but that doesn't mean someone will give them to you. It takes hard work and effort every day to make the choices that will allow you to live the life you want to live. Remember: it's your life and only you can take responsibility for it. The first step is getting to know yourself again and being able to accept that you're not perfect, and that neither do you need to be. Extend the hand of friendship to yourself, learn to forgive yourself for the mistakes you make and remind yourself of the good things you do.

Notes to myself

16

Keep perspective

Being good to yourself

Change involves actively choosing a healthier and more positive path, step by step. Nothing can replace the benefits of doing the work, gaining self-awareness and integrating mindfulness into your life. Not only does it realign your mind with your body and reduce your levels of stress, it also reinforces your own message to yourself that you are responsible for this invaluable asset – your life. It reminds you that you have choice, freedom and opportunity and a resilience on which you can rely whenever life feels harsh or unkind. You cannot control the future but you can look after yourself so that you can withstand even the worst of life, as well as enjoy the pleasures it can bring.

Life without depression and anxiety

It's quite difficult thinking about what you would be like, as a person, if you didn't feel anxious or depressed. It's easy to say that you'll be happy, go places and do things, but it's worth thinking about this at a much deeper level. What would you, as a person, be like? What would you leave behind, need to forfeit or relinquish if you were no longer anxious or depressed? How would you manage all aspects of yourself and your life without those familiar feelings? Would others respond to you in the same way? Do you fear you'll be left to fend for yourself? Would you be able to meet those ideals you've created of yourself without your anxiety and depression? These are important things to consider as they can help bridge the unconscious, or unformulated, fears you might be carrying around with you that can sabotage your moving beyond your mood and all that comes with it.

Change is frightening as you know your mental landscape so well that even considering a shift to something new can seem terrifying. You know how to feel bad about yourself, how to be critical and harsh, how to stand on the edge of life and watch others having a nice time and feel that regret. What can't be forgotten is that the familiarity of your sadness and fear, your anger and insecurity is just that: familiar – that old worn slipper you'd like to replace but that knows the shape of your foot so well. It's the same with your emotions. You get drawn back to what you know because it's known so well, not only emotionally but also neurologically within those neuronal pathways.

Once more, what wires together fires together, so if you feel bad about yourself and tell yourself that in so many ways, each day it will fire together with the neurons and form a pathway in your brain. With time, you won't even need to say anything negative to yourself but simply have a fleeting response for your brain to jump on to that pathway and set it in motion. You get on that track to London even if that isn't where you want to go (see Chapter 9).

This is one of the reasons mindfulness practices are so important to do on a regular basis, because they help you to develop new pathways and to refocus the attention away from the old one and strengthen the newer one until that one becomes familiar. It's not only in the meditations that you're doing this, but each time you start along a track of 'I'm useless, horrible and awful', you can stop, step off that track and put yourself on another more helpful one. The more you know yourself, the more sense mindfulness will make in your life.

Something worth noting is that depression and anger are closely linked and can be the flip side of each other. When there is anger that feels unmanageable, that can't be expressed or reasoned, then it's sometimes easier to turn it in on yourself as depression. For example, if you are angry with a parent about something from the past but you're not allowed to say anything, what happens to that anger? It frequently bubbles up and can feel as if it's going to overwhelm you or be destructive to the other person, so the safer way to manage it is by turning it in on yourself in the form of depression, and sometimes it even takes on the shape of telling yourself what a terrible person you are or simply feeling exhausted by the unexpressed anger that can find no other way out.

Anxiety can be about your own fears about what you might do if you put your anger out into the world. Then what would happen? Would you be destructive and damaging to someone? If so, then the safer route is to turn it around and for you to see the world as being a frightening, fearful place rather than yourself as someone who could create fear or damage. These are only examples, but what is necessary is to look beyond the emotion and to know what's driving it. Medication can tame the feelings but not make sense of them or sort them out in any way.

Gratitude

A way of viewing gratitude is from the perspective of recognizing and acknowledging, with grace, what you have in your life. Gratitude can increase determination, attention, enthusiasm and energy in adults and adolescents,[1,2] it has a direct impact for people with chronic pain on improved sleep and decreased depression (the improved sleep lessens anxiety),[3] and not only is it strongly correlated with well-being but it has the potential to improve well-being through practising it.[4] Even in the worst of times there are threads of things that can be seen as decent, adequate or good. When you view your life, for all that it is, with a sense of grace and gratefulness, it helps to ground you in life's nuances. Not every minute of every day is filled with anxiety or depression, nor is each moment a fight for survival. Inevitably, if you monitor each day you'll get to recognize that some parts of the day are more difficult or easier, that some days are better than others and that there may even be some weeks that are more pleasant. By having a willingness to see your life with eyes that can see the good and the harsh and feel a sense of thankfulness for the good, no matter how small, you help yourself to keep perspective. A smile from someone, a few minutes of laugher with a friend, a hug from a partner, a kind gesture from a stranger, a warm bath, a comfortable bed, food in your belly – there's never a shortage of things for which to be grateful, and a few moments of acknowledging them helps you to recognize that the harsh and the good co-exist, just as the easier and trickier parts of yourself co-exist within you but all in one unit, you. Keep a daily or weekly note of things for which you are grateful.

Compassion and kindness

Linked with gratitude is compassion, a feeling and showing of tenderness and softness towards suffering. Somehow it seems easier to feel compassion for the suffering of others and their foibles than your own. In some ways the idea of showing compassion towards yourself is removed from our social and cultural norms. It's associated with religious figures who do good or tell us to do good, those saintly people who help the most vulnerable in forsaken and devastated areas. The thrust of modern media messages is a far cry from this, promoting denial, avoidance, self-centredness and individual pursuit and gain at all costs.

Within this context, to find and develop that knowing that you too are allowed to be shown kindness and softness, by yourself, to yourself, is something that may need to be learnt. Without it, you will have little to act as a buffer when you make mistakes or fail to meet your harsh expectations.

Notes to myself

17

Take care

Managing expectations

True happiness and fulfilment does not mean that everything is always bright and shiny. It's about accepting that life can be difficult at times, knowing that during those times you have the resourcefulness to manage them and the ability to enjoy the better times in full, even those fleeting moments.

Depression and anxiety can affect your life on every level, and it may take time before you begin to notice the benefits of changing your mindset, getting to know yourself and doing the mindfulness practices. It should take time, as this isn't about flipping a switch or changing an outfit. This isn't a competition – but there can be a winner if you keep at it. It's not going to be what fits for everyone but if it is right for you, then keep going, one foot in front of the other.

Setting boundaries

You may find that making time to complete the practices is difficult or that your family do not give you the time alone you need. It's up to you to set boundaries in order to get what you need from the practices. Try explaining to your family, friends or partner the basics of what mindfulness is and why you want to do the practice; they may well be interested in it and it could be a way into talking more openly about your feelings of anxiety or depression with loved ones. Put aside some time each day for yourself, whether that is 20 minutes for a Mindful Awareness meditation or 5 minutes to make a cup of tea mindfully or sit quietly – it all counts. You may also want to try some of the practices with friends or family – children are naturally mindful, so they enjoy the practices (which can be adapted to suit their age), and it's a lovely way to spend time together.

Mindfulness practice: Self-care Meditation

This meditation is a starting point for developing a kind and caring attitude towards yourself. Sit quietly in any position that is comfortable for you and take a few mindful breaths. Repeat the following phrases to yourself:

- May I be happy and healthy.
- May I accept myself for all that I am.
- May I be free from pain and suffering.

Repeat these phrases a number of times, even when it feels difficult. When we're anxious or depressed we can start to doubt that we're worthy of love or that we deserve to be happy. These are just thoughts however; we don't need to latch on to them. Everyone is deserving of love and happiness and you can start to cultivate a sense of kindness and care towards yourself. Change the wording to suit your own ideas of generosity, kindness and care towards yourself.

Taking care

Take care of yourself as you start to move forwards with your life. Acknowledge that you are building a more engaged future with every building block of 'now'.

Even if your plans don't work out, you can't fail as long as you're making the choices that are right for you.

The chances are that you will make mistakes and that you will struggle at times, because life is never simple or easy. The difference now will be that you have the resources and the strength to make your own decisions, take responsibility for your life and to be alive with each moment. You need to be your own best friend, your own champion who understands yourself, learns from your life and who can be respectful and kind towards yourself and others. Most of all, you can maintain your balance and your dignity, no matter what life throws at you.

There is no end with mindfulness. It's about recognizing and absorbing the awareness that life is impermanent and transient, that things shift and change because that's life, and about managing your life using this mindset of mindfulness, the practices, gratitude and compassion, one day at a time and one breath at a time.

Cultivating a bountiful mind

The whole idea behind this book is about developing a mindset that goes far beyond your cognitions or thoughts. It's about cultivating your bountiful mind, which is far greater than your brain functions, thoughts or processes. Your bountiful mind encompasses all of you, your personal and individual abilities to think, feel, love, be aware, sense, imagine, create, know and respond. It's your conscious and unconscious, your individuality and your connectedness to others. It's your greater, fuller and deeper awareness of you and all that you've incorporated into it from being a human being, having experiences and breathing in all the life around you.

It is this mind, this substantial, plentiful mind, that you must draw on to balance out the damaging effects of your ongoing depression and anxiety and your struggles with understanding and managing your distress.

Courage is needed to manage life, to learn and to hold steadfast when the seas are rough and hope seems distant. Without courage, gratitude and compassion you'll be left afloat on those harsh waves with little to hold on to. We aren't born with courage and resilience, and self-compassion is often squeezed out of us from an early age, being seen as an excuse for lack of self-discipline.

Courage means being loyal to yourself even if others aren't, stepping up to yourself and your life. It takes commitment, hard work and a shifting of beliefs because life is tough and we often aren't given the tools or taught the skills on how to manage it. The fact that you are alive means that there will be suffering, pain, fear, anger and many other situations and emotions. If you start from the baseline of thinking life is easy and gentle and all will be well, then you start from a disadvantage as any reality of pain and suffering will be regarded as something out of the ordinary, unlucky or rare. If you recognize that the very fact of being alive and all that comes with it is sometimes wonderful, sometimes ordinary and sometimes awful, then you don't set yourself up to believe that you're a failure or that you have an unlucky life. Part of what helps to get through all the changes in life is to have a strong internal compass that shows you when you're going off course, which direction you're heading in and how to get back on track. Others can help you develop this, but only you can cultivate it within yourself – and if you do, it will be the one thing you can always hold on to, no matter where you are, how you are feeling or what is happening in your life.

Live your life one breath at a time.

Notes

1 Connecting the dots

1   Halliwell, E., Main, L. and Richardson, C. (2007), *The Fundamental Facts: The Latest Facts and Figures on Mental Health*, London: Mental Health Foundation, <www.mentalhealth.org.uk/content/assets/PDF/publications/fundamental_facts_2007.pdf?view–Standard>.

2 Anxiety, depression and mindfulness

1   Bracha, H. S. (2004), 'Freeze, Flight, Fight, Fright, Faint: Adaptationist Perspectives on the Acute Stress Response Spectrum', *CNS Spectrums* 9(9), pp. 679–85.

2   Allen, N., Chambers, R., Knight, W., Blashki, G., Ciechomski, L., Hassed, C., Gullone, E., McNab, C. and Meadows, G. (2006), 'Mindfulness-based Psychotherapies: A Review of Conceptual Foundations, Empirical Evidence and Practical Considerations', *Australian and New Zealand Journal of Psychiatry* 40(4), pp. 285–94.

3 Facts, figures and you

1   <www.who.int/mediacentre/factsheets/fs369/en>.

2   <www.mentalhealth.org.uk/help-information/mental-health-statistics>.

3   <www.adaa.org/understanding-anxiety/depression>.

4   <www.mentalhealth.org.uk/help-information/mental-health-statistics>.

5   <www.mentalhealth.org.uk/help-information/mental-health-statistics>.

6   <www.adaa.org/understanding-anxiety/depression>.

7   <wwwwho.int/mediacentre/factsheets/fs369/en>.

8   <www.save.org/index.cfm?fuseaction=home.viewPage&page_id= 705D5DF4-055B-F1EC 3F66462866FCB4E6>.

9   <www.who.int/mediacentre/news/releases/2014/suicide-prevention-report/en>.

10   Rezek, C. A. (2002), 'Depression Across the Lifespan', doctoral thesis, London: City University.

11 Wiech, K. and Tracey, I., 'The Influence of Negative Emotions on Pain: Behavioral Effects and Neural Mechanisms', *Neuroimage* 47(3), pp. 987–94.

12 <www.hse.gov.uk/statistics/causdis/stress/stress.pdf>.

13 <www.cbi.org.uk/media/2150120/cbi-pfizer_absence___workplace_ health_2013.pdf>.

14 <www.save.org/index.cfm?fuseaction=home.viewPage&page_id=705D5D F4-055B-F1EC-3F66462866FCB4E6>; <www.nimh.nih.gov/index.shtml>.

15 <www.adaa.org/understanding-anxiety/depression>.

16 <www.nimh.nih.gov/index.shtml>.

17 <www.mentalhealth.org.uk/help-information/mental-health-statistics>.

18 Office of National Statistics (2014). *Suicides in the United Kingdom: 2012 Registrations*, London: ONS.

19 <www.who.int/mediacentre/news/releases/2014/suicide-prevention-report/en>.

20 <www.who.int/mediacentre/factsheets/fs369/en>.

21 <www.who.int/mediacentre/news/releases/2014/suicide-prevention-report/en>; <www.who.int/mediacentre/factsheets/fs369/en>.

6 No magic pills

1 Grossman, P., Niemann, L., Schmidt, S. and Walach, H. (2004), 'Mindfulness-based Stress Reduction and Health Benefits: A Meta-analysis', *Journal of Psychosomatic Research* 57(1), pp. 35–44.

2 Gotink, R. A., Chu, P., Busschbach, J. J., Benson, H., Fricchione, G. L. and Hunink, M. G. (2015), 'Standardised Mindfulness-based Interventions in Healthcare: An Overview of Systematic Reviews and Meta-analyses of RCTs', *PLoS One*, Doi: 10.1371/journal.pone.0124344.

3 Zeidan, F., Johnson, S. K., Diamond, B. J., David, Z. and Goolkasian, P. (2010), 'Mindfulness Meditation Improves Cognition: Evidence of Brief Mental Training', *Consciousness and Cognition* 19(2), pp. 597–605.

4 Reibel, D. K., Greeson, J. M., Brainard, G. C. and Rosenzweig, S. (2001), 'Mindfulness-based Stress Reduction and Health-related Quality of Life in a Heterogeneous Patient Population', *General Hospital Psychiatry* 23(4), pp. 183–92.

5 Guardino, C. M., Dunkel Schetter, C., Bower, J. E., Lu, M. C. and Smalley, S. L. (2014), 'Randomised Controlled Pilot Trial of Mindfulness Training for Stress Reduction During Pregnancy', *Psychological Health* 29(3), pp. 70–7.

6 Davidson, R. J., Kabat-Zinn, J., Schumacher, J., Rosenkranz, M., Muller, D., Santorelli, S. F., Urbanowski F., Harrington A., Bonus K. and Sheridan, J. F. (2003), 'Alterations in Brain and Immune Function Produced by Mindfulness Meditation', *Psychosomatic Medicine* 65(4), pp. 564–70.

7   Howell, A. J., Digdon, N. L., Buro, K. and Sheptycki, A. R. (2008), 'Relations Among Mindfulness, Well-being, and Sleep', *Personality and Individual Differences* 45(8), pp. 773–7.

8   Beauchemin, J., Hutchins, T. L. and Patterson, F. (2008), 'Mindfulness Meditation may Lessen Anxiety, Promote Social Skills, and Improve Academic Performance among Adolescents with Learning Disabilities', *Journal of Evidence-Based Complementary and Alternative Medicine* 13(1), pp. 34–45.

9   Singh, N. N., Lancioni, G. E., Winton, A. S., Singh, J., Curtis, W. J., Wahler, R. G. and McAleavey, K. M. (2007), 'Mindful Parenting Decreases Aggression and Increases Social Behavior in Children with Developmental Disabilities', *Behavior Modification* 31(6), pp. 749–71.

10   Glomb, T. M., Duffy, M. K., Bono, J. E. and Yang, T. (2011), 'Mindfulness at Work', *Research in Personnel and Human Resources Management* 30, pp. 115–57.

11   Witkiewitz, K., Marlatt, G. A. and Walker, D. (2005), 'Mindfulness-Based Relapse Prevention for Alcohol and Substance Use Disorders', *Journal of Cognitive Psychotherapy* 19(3), pp. 211–28.

12   Follette, V., Palm, K. M. and Pearson, A. N. (2006), 'Mindfulness and Trauma: Implications for Treatment', *Journal of Rational-Emotive and Cognitive-Behavior Therapy* 24(1), pp. 45–61.

13   Bernstein, A., Tanay, G. and Vujanovic, A. A. (2011), 'Concurrent Relations between Mindful Attention and Awareness and Psychopathology among Trauma-Exposed Adults: Preliminary Evidence of Transdiagnostic Resilience', *Journal of Cognitive Psychotherapy* 25(2), pp. 99–113.

14   <www.apa.org/monitor/2015/03/cover-mindfulness.aspx>.

15   Kuyken, W. et al. (2015), 'Effectiveness and Cost-Effectiveness of Mindfulness-based Cognitive Therapy Compared with Maintenance Antidepressant Treatment in the Prevention of Depressive Relapse or Recurrence (PREVENT): A Randomised Controlled Trial', *The Lancet* 386(9988), pp. 63–73.

16   Goldacre, B. (2009), *Bad Science*, London: Harper Perennial.

17   Goldacre, B. (2013), *Bad Pharma*, London: Fourth Estate.

18   Kuyken et al., 'Effectiveness and Cost-effectiveness of Mindfulness-based Cognitive Therapy'.

/ Connections

1   Brown, K. W. and Ryan, R. M. (2003), 'The Benefits of Being Present: Mindfulness and its Role in Psychological Well-being', *Journal of Personality and Social Psychology* 84(4), pp. 822–48.

2   Haug, T. T., Mykletun, A. and Dahl, A. A. (2004), 'The Association between Anxiety, Depression, and Somatic Symptoms in a Large Population: The HUNT-II Study', *Psychosomatic Medicine* 66(6), pp. 845–51.

3   Borrell-Carrió, F., Suchman, A. L. and Epstein, R. M. (2004), 'The Biopsychosocial Model 25 Years Later: Principles, Practice, and Scientific Inquiry', *The Annals of Family Medicine* 2(6), pp. 576–82.

4   Nair, S., Sagar, M., Sollers, J., Consedine, N., Broadbent, E. (2015), 'Do Slumped and Upright Postures Affect Stress Responses? A Randomized Trial', *Health Psychology* 34(6), pp. 632–41.

8 The development of self

1   Roberts, J. E., Gotlib, I. H. and Kassel, J. D. (1996), 'Adult Attachment Security and Symptoms of Depression: The Mediating Roles of Dysfunctional Attitudes and Low Self-esteem', *Journal of Personality and Social Psychology* 70(2), pp. 310–20.

2   Styron, T. and Janoff-Bulman, R. (1997), 'Childhood Attachment and Abuse: Long-term Effects on Adult Attachment, Depression, and Conflict Resolution', *Child Abuse and Neglect* 21(10), pp. 1015–23.

3   Bifulco, A., Kwon, J., Jacobs, C., Moran, P. M., Bunn, A. and Beer, N. (2006), 'Adult Attachment Style as Mediator Between Childhood Neglect/Abuse and Adult Depression and Anxiety', *Social Psychiatry and Psychiatric Epidemiology* 41(10), pp. 796–805.

4   Cramer, P. (2000), 'Defense Mechanisms in Psychology Today: Further Processes for Adaptation', *American Psychologist* 55(6), pp. 637–46.

9 Anxiety and depression in context

1   Yehuda, R., Resnick, H., Kahana, B. and Giller, E. L. (1993), 'Long-lasting Hormonal Alterations to Extreme Stress in Humans: Normative or Maladaptive?', *Psychosomatic Medicine* 55(3), pp. 287–97.

2   Davidson, R. J., Jackson, D. C. and Kalin, N. H. (2000), 'Emotion, Plasticity, Context, and Regulation: Perspectives from Affective Neuroscience', *Psychological Bulletin* 126(6), pp. 890–909.

3   Stein, D. J. (2006), 'Advances in Understanding the Anxiety Disorders: The Cognitive-affective Neuroscience of "False Alarms"', *Annals of Clinical Psychiatry* 18(3), pp. 173–82.

4   Nutt, D. J. (2008), 'Relationship of Neurotransmitters to the Symptoms of Major Depressive Disorder', *Journal of Clinical Psychiatry* 69 Suppl. E1, pp. 4–7.

5   Pyszczynski, T., Hamilton, J. C., Herring, F. H. and Greenberg, J. (1989), 'Depression, Self-focused Attention, and the Negative Memory Bias', *Journal of Personality and Social Psychology* 57(2), pp. 351–7.

6   Clarke, P., Macleod, C. and Shirazee, N. (2008), 'Prepared for the Worst: Readiness to Acquire Threat Bias and Susceptibility to Elevate Trait Anxiety', *Emotion* 8(1), pp. 47–57.

7   Joormann, J., Dkane, M. and Gotlib, I. H. (2006), 'Adaptive and Maladaptive Components of Rumination? Diagnostic Specificity and Relation to Depressive Biases', *Behavior Therapy* 37(3), pp. 269–80.

8   Rutter, M. (1985), 'Resilience in the Face of Adversity: Protective Factors and Resistance to Psychiatric Disorder', *British Journal of Psychiatry* 147(1), pp. 598–611.

9   Shapiro, S. L., Carlson, L. E., Astin, J. A. and Freedman, B. (2006), 'Mechanisms of Mindfulness', *Journal of Clinical Psychology* 62(3), pp. 373–86.

10 The stress response

1   Jansen, A. S., Van Nguyen, X. V., Karpitskiy, V., Mettenleiter, T. C. and Loewy, A. D. (1995), 'Central Command Neurons of the Sympathetic Nervous System: Basis of the Fight-or-Flight Response', *Science* 270(5236), pp. 644–6.

2   Eilam, D. (2005), 'Die Hard: A Blend of Freezing and Fleeing as a Dynamic Defense – Implications for the Control of Defensive Behavior', *Neuroscience and Biobehavioral Reviews* 29(8), pp. 1181–91.

3   Segerstrom, S. C. and Miller, G. E. (2004), 'Psychological Stress and the Human Immune System: A Meta-Analytic Study of 30 Years of Inquiry', *Psychological Bulletin* 130(4), pp. 601–30.

4   Gardner-Nix, J. (2010), *The Mindfulness Solution to Pain: Step-by-Step Techniques for Chronic Pain Management*, Oakland, CA: New Harbinger.

5   McGonagle, K. A. and Kessler, R. C. (1990), 'Chronic stress, acute stress, and depressive symptoms', *American Journal of Community Psychology* 18(5), 681–706.

6   Gardner-Nix, *Mindfulness Solution to Pain*.

7   Gold, P. W., Goodwin, F. K. and Chrousos, G. P. (1988), 'Clinical and Biochemical Manifestations of Depression: Relation to the Neurobiology of Stress (2)', *New England Journal of Medicine* 319(7), pp. 413–20.

8   Schmidt, N. B., Lerew, D. R. and Jackson, R. J. (1997), 'The Role of Anxiety Sensitivity in the Pathogenesis of Panic: Prospective Evaluation

of Spontaneous Panic Attacks During Acute Stress', *Journal of Abnormal Psychology* 106(3), pp. 355–64.

11 Effects of mindfulness on the brain

1 Davidson, R. J., Kabat-Zinn, J., Schumacher, J., Rosenkranz, M., Muller, D., Santorelli, S. F. and Sheridan, J. F. (2003), 'Alterations in Brain and Immune Function Produced by Mindfulness Meditation', *Psychosomatic Medicine* 65(4), pp. 564–70.

2 Davidson et al., 'Alterations in Brain and Immune Function'.

3 Hölzel, B. K., Carmody, J., Vangel, M., Congleton, C., Yerramsetti, S. M., Gard, T. and Lazar, S. W. (2011), 'Mindfulness Practice Leads to Increases in Regional Brain Gray Matter Density', *Psychiatry Research: Neuroimaging* 191(1), pp. 36–43.

4 Coffey, K. A., Hartman, M. and Fredrickson, B. L. (2010), 'Deconstructing Mindfulness and Constructing Mental Health: Understanding Mindfulness and its Mechanisms of Action', *Mindfulness* 1(4), pp. 235–53.

5 Pressley, M., Wood, E., Woloshyn, V. E., Martin, V., King, A. and Menke, D. (1992), 'Encouraging Mindful use of Prior Knowledge: Attempting to Construct Explanatory Answers Facilitates Learning', *Educational Psychologist* 27(1), pp. 91–109.

6 Heeren, A., Van Broeck, N. and Philippot, P. (2009), 'The effects of mindfulness on executive processes and autobiographical memory specificity', *Behaviour Research and Therapy* 47(5), pp. 403–9.

7 Brown, K. W. and Ryan, R. M. (2003), 'The Benefits of Being Present: Mindfulness and its Role in Psychological Well-being', *Journal of Personality and Social Psychology* 84(4), pp. 822–48.

8 Allen, N., Chambers, R., Knight, W., Blashki, G., Ciechomski, L., Hassed, C., Gullone, E., McNab, C. and Meadows, G. (2006), 'Mindfulness-based Psychotherapies: A Review of Conceptual Foundations, Empirical Evidence and Practical Considerations', *Australian and New Zealand Journal of Psychiatry* 40(4), pp. 285–94.

13 Why me?

1 Hayes, A. M. and Feldman, G. (2004), 'Clarifying the Construct of Mindfulness in the Context of Emotion Regulation and the Process of Change in Therapy' *Clinical Psychology: Science and Practice* 11(3), pp. 255–62.

16 Keep perspective

1   Emmons, R. A. and McCullough, M. E. (2003), 'Counting Blessings versus Burdens: An Experimental Investigation of Gratitude and Subjective Well-being in Daily Life', *Journal of Personality and Social Psychology* 84(2), pp. 377–89.

2   Froh, J. J., Sefick, W. J. and Emmons, R. A. (2008), 'Counting Blessings in Early Adolescents: An Experimental Study of Gratitude and Subjective Well-being', *Journal of School Psychology* 46(2), pp. 213–33.

3   Ng, M. Y. and Wong, W. S. (2013), 'The Differential Effects of Gratitude and Sleep on Psychological Distress in Patients with Chronic Pain', *Journal of Health Psychology* 18(2), pp. 263–271.

4   Wood, A. M., Froh, J. J. and Geraghty, A. W. (2010), 'Gratitude and Well-being: A Review and Theoretical Integration', *Clinical Psychology Review* 30(7), pp. 890–905.